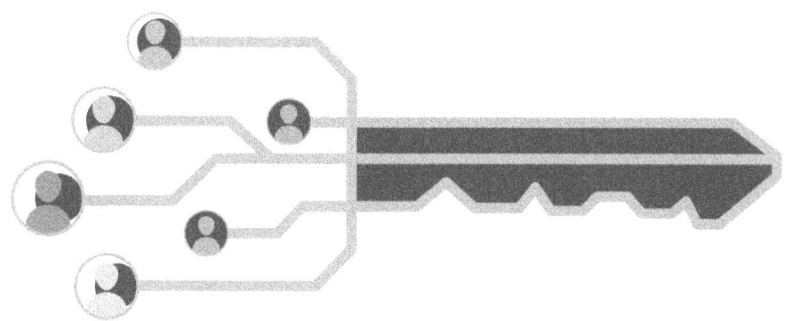

Data-Driven Healthcare

From information to impact in the digital age

CHRIS MAY

Data-Driven Healthcare

ISBN 978-1-917490-08-5

eISBN 978-1-917490-09-2

Published in 2026 by Right Book Press

Manufactured by
Sue Richardson Associates Ltd.
Studio 6,
9, Marsh Street
Bristol
BS1 4AA

info@therightbookcompany.com

EU Safety Representative
eucomply OÜ
Parnu mnt 139b-14
11317 Tallinn
Estonia

hello@eucompliancepartner.com
+33 756 90241

© Chris May

The right of Chris May to be identified as the author of this work has been asserted in accordance with the Copyright, Designs and Patents Act 1988.

A CIP record of this book is available from the British Library.

All rights reserved. No part of this book may be reproduced, stored in a retrieval system, or transmitted in any form or by any means, electronic, mechanical, photocopying, recording or otherwise, without the prior written permission of the copyright holder.

There are few voices in the industry I take as seriously as Chris May's. In this clear and informed book, he gives us an overview of the current tech landscape as well as highlighting the key themes that are central to shaping its future. His approach is grounded in public expectation, informed by what's technologically possible, and acutely aware of the unique challenges facing healthcare services.
   – Dr Ben Allen, GP partner & medical director

A refreshing and humane approach to artificial intelligence, one that appreciates the vital collaboration between patient, doctor and software. Standardising and personalisation might seem like polar opposites, but May makes it crystal clear why we do better with both.
   – Margaret Heffernan, CEO & author

This book offers fascinating insight at a time when harnessing the power of data in healthcare has never been more important – or more possible.
   – Rachel Heggart, senior project manager, NHS England

A welcome provocation on how we can harness data and digital innovations to better personalise care. This book is useful for all in the healthcare community, as it shows how we can become more patient-centric by using insights gleaned from data to predict needs and prevent harm.
   – Tara Donnelly, former chief digital officer, NHS England
     & founder, www.Digital.Care

Data-Driven Healthcare paints a compelling picture of the vastly untapped potential for using the data already available within the healthcare system to dramatically influence and improve patient outcomes. Blissfully jargon free and wide ranging in its scope, it is a comprehensive primer for anyone interested in delving into the world of health data.
   – Lucy Ellis-Brookes, deputy director in data & analytics,
     NHS England

Chris May sets out the path for a data-driven and patient-centric healthcare ecosystem that makes the most out of the latest advances in technology. A valuable read for clinicians, managers and investors alike.

– Yasemin Arik, healthcare investor & partner, G Square Capital

Chris May articulates the vision many of us in digital health share but often struggle to express: patient-centred, outcome-driven care built on interoperable, intelligent systems. He makes a clear, compelling case for moving from data collection to data use, and issues a timely call to action for everyone involved in healthcare. We owe it to our clinicians, patients and the NHS to get the full value from the available data to drive better outcomes for all.

– Nick Hopkinson, executive coach for digital leaders
 & healthcare CIO

Full of insight, history and lessons to apply to the future, this book can become a guiding light for healthcare professionals. The knowledge and experiences that Chris May shares will help you lead the way in a new healthcare delivery, one that is data driven and delivers insight for all.

– Richard Corbridge, former healthcare CIO, UK & Ireland
 & fellow of the British Computer Society

With the vast majority of patient data remaining unused, this book is a call to arms, making the case for how this data can and should be used to revolutionise patient care and improve outcomes.

– Dr Michelle Tempest, senior partner, Candesic & author of
 Big Brain Revolution: Artificial Intelligence – Spy or Saviour?

An illuminating and informed portrayal of the staggering promise of healthcare technology advancement. Chris May clearly articulates how embracing the better use of data can achieve truly patient-centric healthcare.

– Hemavli Bali, director of healthcare M&A, Clearwater
 International

Contents

Preface	1
1 Healthcare in the information age	11
2 The challenge for healthcare	15
3 Emerging technology trends	23
4 The impact of AI	61
5 The rise of data in healthcare	65
6 The care record	73
7 Data-driven healthcare	85
8 Key themes	95
9 Clinical records – the next generation	125
10 Challenges to adoption	131
11 Conclusion – the future is bright	145
References	147
Acknowledgements	151
About the author	153

To all past, present and future employees of Mayden who have given up a portion of their lives to support clinicians to provide the very best care for their patients.

Preface

This is a book about data – healthcare data – and the digital revolution taking place today that will enable us to unlock its full value. While this book is aimed primarily at healthcare professionals across the globe, I am aware that there is an intrinsic problem: the majority of those I am addressing here either have no access to digital tools, or if they do, given the choice, would still largely prefer pen and paper.

Most clinicians just want to treat the patient in front of them, to bring to bear all their many years of training and experience, in combination with latest diagnostic techniques that science has provided and to offer a reasonable choice of evidence-based options for treatment. Those I grew up alongside were not particularly interested in what the patient thought, or in the opinions of the patient's friends or family, and would not have cared what Google said or about anyone the social media platforms might have dragged up as self-appointed experts with little or no training.

Today's clinicians are highly trained professionals who rely on their knowledge and skills to make better and better decisions for the patients who present to them, albeit operating in a landscape of ever-expanding alternative, traditional, Eastern and functional (root cause-based) medicine narratives that compete with established (Western) protocols. They will seek a second opinion if need be. They will increasingly make those decisions as part of a multi-disciplinary team where a variety of expertise is gathered to look at a problem holistically. And increasingly they will consult Google, PubMed, etc, and consider evidence and suggestions provided by their patients.

What they won't do, in that moment, is gather all the intelligence available from the records of all the other patients around the world presenting with similar profiles, symptoms and diagnoses, and review what treatments they are having and what outcomes are being achieved. Why not? The answer to that question is complex and speaks to key themes that I will be revisiting throughout this book. But it isn't because it's technically impossible.

When my mother fell ill in 1986, I was 100 miles away, happily designing and constructing chocolate production lines in the factory that inspired Roald Dahl's famous story. My job (if you can call it that – I got to play with the latest computer technology all day and eat vast quantities of my favourite food for free) was essentially to automate what had historically been manual tasks. In other words, to replace unreliable, fallible people – sometimes presenting dubious work ethics – with digital control systems.

On one particular automation project – codenamed 'Aubergine' to prevent the competition's industrial espionage teams guessing what we were up to (another name for aubergine is *eggplant*) – 50 people were replaced with 20 and a plethora of computers. The latter set about monitoring temperatures, pressures, humidity, viscosity, conveyor belt sensors, etc, constantly adjusting a wide range of parameters to ensure that every resulting chocolate egg – and I'm talking about a million each day – was of a consistent high quality. The former were primarily there to watch a myriad of flashing lights and clean up any mess when it all went wrong. Which, in those early days of commissioning a new plant, it did with frustrating regularity. Most of the sensors were designed to stop the plant from running if anything went out of range. All that data, captured in real time, just to ensure that every chocolate bar that came out of that factory was nothing less than perfect. And they were. Perfect. Every one of them.

My mother didn't come out of hospital perfect. In fact, she didn't come out of hospital at all. After an initial misdiagnosis and a prescribed treatment regimen designed to cure what she didn't have, the doctors eventually found a malignant tumour. They operated and believed they had been successful in removing the cancer. But my mother never recovered from the surgery, gradually deteriorated while those around her watched helplessly and passed away. To this day I don't really know the full facts surrounding my mother's death. I never saw a published diagnosis naming the type of cancer she had, or where the stated tumour was located, or why she failed to recover from the surgery when all expectations at the time were otherwise, or what, given that the tumour was completely removed, was her ultimate cause of death. At the time I didn't think to ask; it wasn't going to change anything. But years later, while working on a national project to assess the readiness of cancer services across England to provide care to an appropriate standard, I discovered that the hospital in which she died had not done so well. Its scores were lower than comparable hospitals pretty much across the board. If the genesis of this book could be traced to any one time, it was in that moment.

You might have noticed that in one paragraph I am making chocolate and in the next I'm reviewing cancer services. How did that happen? Once project 'Aubergine' had finally settled into what was to become normal running mode, I left the chocolate factory to extend my skills and experience into other areas. As an engineer specialising in manufacturing systems, I found there was a myriad of outlets for my talents – but which to choose? In the end I took up a position as a senior fellow at the University of Cambridge, where the responsibilities of my day job still gave me plenty of time to explore other avenues. My salary was generously funded by Rio Tinto, a multinational, cross-sector conglomerate, who were only too happy for me to set about problem-solving across their portfolio of companies while I simultaneously managed student projects in a number of other organisations on behalf of the university's postgraduate Advanced Course in Design, Manufacture and Management.

One of these projects was established in Papworth Hospital, an internationally renowned cardiothoracic centre located just outside Cambridge. Papworth was a revelation. Its dedicated team of clinicians were pioneering new cardiothoracic techniques, particularly in the area of heart and lung transplantation – but the whole place ran on a handful of low-specification PCs. And there was absolutely no data in sight. The hospital was aware of this but technologically speaking it was run as a satellite of the larger general hospital up the road, which consumed all the local IT skills and resources.

I was fascinated. Compared to the manufacturing environments I was used to, Papworth seemed like a backwater. Consequently, the potential to really make a difference was huge. I soon realised that this state of affairs – management by lack of information – was reflected to a greater or lesser extent in hospitals up and down the country. I offered some of my time to Papworth for free and they finally caved in and offered me a job. I accepted and my transition into healthcare was complete. Now I had a new career and a mission: to bring the level of information technology used in the NHS to that enjoyed by manufacturing industries. All by myself. Easy.

When I say 'all by myself' that clearly isn't true. So why say it? Because in those early years I was the only healthcare manager I knew with a technical background, moreover an engineer and one specialising in manufacturing systems. Most of my colleagues trained in the humanities and many of the more senior managers were ex-armed forces. That was how the NHS ran then. In retrospect I shouldn't have been surprised. If you were a talented engineer, why would you choose to work in the health service? I had quickly realised that manufacturing had nothing to learn from the health sector; it was all the other way round. I wasn't special in any sense that manufacturing would recognise, but in the NHS I found I was fairly unique – just because I thought differently about information and data.

Over the next decade, my career was wide and varied. After leaving Papworth, I continued to apply data analytics to a variety of local and national problems until I was fortunate enough to join an embryonic management consultancy that would eventually become the most successful healthcare-focused consultancy in the country. The six years I spent there gave me access to the full range of problems facing the healthcare sector and I spent most of that time working on a number of new hospital developments and whole-system service reviews up and down the country. But my passion remained in the data – certainly not the politics – and in 2000 I founded Mayden as a boutique healthcare analytics business aiming to take advantage of a newfangled thing called the internet, essentially returning to my roots and what I thought then was my prime motivation for being in healthcare in the first place, namely to surface the gold that was hidden in the vast ocean of patient data.

One year in, Mayden was commissioned to provide analytics and consultancy support to the newly formed cancer network covering north central London. Though I had worked on many hospital-based projects that had naturally included cancer services, this was actually the first time I was up close and personal with the disease that had taken my uncle and my mother, both at an early age. On the back of the 1995 national Calman–Hine review of cancer services, significant resources were suddenly being put into cancer care in a serious attempt to bring the NHS in England in line with cancer services around the globe. All the data suggested we were falling behind and survival rates were relatively poor. Furthermore, within the country there was clearly a postcode lottery at work and how well you did with cancer was reflected in where you lived, something which was an anathema to the population at large and which the media had rightly jumped on. The first task was to take the temperature of cancer service provision across the country and assess just how well services were actually performing against what Calman–Hine considered to be appropriate standards for providing quality care.

Here, then, is how the NHS initially responded: a manual of cancer services was printed and posted out to every cancer team in every hospital in the country, together with thousands of pages of self-assessment forms tailored to each type of cancer. The assessments took the form of a series of questions to which the answer to each was essentially Yes or No. Each cancer team was given a finite time to complete the paperwork before returning it via the hospital management to their local cancer network. The cancer networks collated all the assessments for hospitals in their patch and then forwarded an aggregated summary and the detailed forms to their local regional office. The regional offices gathered all the assessments from their local cancer networks and forwarded them on to the newly established National Cancer Action Team (NCAT). Once these were in, NCAT was to analyse all the data and produce a report mapping the state of cancer provision nationwide. The exercise from receipt by NCAT to production of the report was earmarked to take six months.

The year was 2001. The internet had been alive and seriously kicking for five years and huge fortunes had been made and lost in the boom and bust which ended the year before. While all that took place, the NHS as a whole had largely ignored the World Wide Web, citing security concerns and pretending it wasn't there. NCAT wasn't unique in this respect; its response to the taking-the-temperature problem simply mirrored similar decisions across the NHS. Yet these problems were crying out for an online solution, one that would enable the data to be captured efficiently and cheaply, put a severe dent in the profits of the photocopier companies and postal services, and where the final report mapping the national state of play would be available in seconds, not months.

With NCAT's support, Mayden built CQuINS, an internet-based system to do just that. Launched in 2003, it was one of the first online applications to be deployed by the NHS nationally and also proved to be possibly the longest serving to date, finally being switched off in March 2019. During its first decade, NCAT, with only a tiny team, presided over a whole-system evolution of our national cancer services, all but removing the postcode lottery and elevating outcomes to those enjoyed by its European and US peers. CQuINS played its part in this, monitoring the steady improvement in service provision with each annual assessment and exposing the results for all to see. There is nothing like peer pressure to stimulate improvement. There is nothing like transparency to drive peer pressure. And there is nothing like data to create transparency.

Just to be clear, underestimating the power of the internet

wasn't exclusive to the NHS. In 2006, Mayden launched a magazine – *Healthcare Today* – summarising healthcare news from around the world. The format was based on a magazine called *The Week*, which had started to gain traction in the UK and later in the US. We thought launching a physical magazine would be a good idea. It wasn't. After 12 issues, the magazine closed but the website that accompanied it rapidly grew to be number one in its category in the UK Google rankings and pulled in thousands of visitors every week.

The day we officially launched the magazine coincided with the genesis of our most successful project to date. We had hired an exhibition stand at the NHS Confederation Conference in Birmingham and were busy handing out free copies of our first edition when we were approached by a clinical psychologist from a London mental health trust. The trust needed a new electronic patient record (EPR) system to be developed to support a pilot project in psychological therapies being run by the Department of Health. None of the systems on the market at the time could deliver what he wanted. The Improving Access to Psychological Therapies programme, IAPT for short, introduced some relatively new concepts to managing patients, namely routine outcome measurement and stepped care pathways, together with a rich, mandated data set that would become one of the cleanest and most complete patient-level data sets in the NHS. Fifteen years on, the newly named NHS Talking Therapies programme has expanded rapidly, both in numbers and geography. The service consists of around 140 adult talking therapy services covering the whole of England, primarily focused on delivering cognitive behavioural therapy (CBT) through a specially trained workforce of psychological wellbeing practitioners (PWPs). Children and young people's (CYP) psychological therapy services began to follow and the model started to attract interest from across the globe.

The application we developed, iaptus, rapidly gained traction in the marketplace and, over the following decade, grew to support two thirds of the adult psychological therapy services across England. It is also in use in Australia and Canada, where organisations there are attempting to introduce the IAPT model into fragmented mental health systems. A special CYP version of the product is also being used to support a range of children's services in both the NHS and UK not-for-profit sectors. At this 15-year point, iaptus holds the records of more than ten million patients, adding more than one million patients and six million clinical contacts each year. It is integrated with more than 30 digital healthcare providers as well as providing access directly into GP systems and a number of other peripheral services such as SMS, hybrid mail and the national NHS Spine. Today, iaptus is branching out into wider clinical areas, supporting services in diabetes remission, cardiovascular disease prevention, gambling addiction and neurodiversity services.

In the almost universally derided industry that is healthcare IT, iaptus scored particularly highly in an independent clinical system usability survey in 2016 (Hoeksma 2016), attracting the most votes from its user base and achieving scores that significantly exceeded those of almost all the other 140 systems in the survey. A follow-up survey in 2022 yielded a similar result (Mayden 2022). Our user support team consistently achieves 99 per cent satisfaction ratings and the iaptus developers gained the accolade of UK Software Development Team of the Year in 2018.

I know we can do more. This, for us, is a journey that is just beginning. An emerging vision of how patient management should be supported by information technology is becoming clearer. The current systems are no longer meeting the needs of clinicians or patients. New entrants to the market are simply replicating the old way of doing things but using new technologies.

The worst failure of our healthcare IT systems has been to suck in vast volumes of data and then do nothing with it. It has been estimated that 97 per cent of patient data that is collected is never used (Moore 2024). This observation sits at the very heart of the challenge we are faced with and emphasises the reason for writing this book.

My mission is both to transform the model for managing patient care and to maximise the benefits from the data that is being collected, along the way exploiting a range of emerging technologies that front-line staff are still only vaguely aware of. If you are a service manager or lead clinician overseeing this clinical activity, this book is primarily for you. Before we – clinicians, managers, IT and data professionals – can all reap the benefits of everything the digisphere has to offer, we first have to set the scene, gain a common understanding of what is both possible and desirable, and then work together – in collaboration – to make it happen.

1 Healthcare in the information age

Data is now the world's most valuable commodity, eclipsing oil, which dominated the world's stock markets for almost a century (Economist 2017). If this is the Information Age, then data is the new oil. Start-up companies which didn't exist five minutes before are finding ever more innovative ways to exploit it and, like oil, the ability of data to flow from its source and achieve global reach is phenomenal. Unlike oil, this can happen to data within seconds.

For a whole variety of reasons, which I will explore later, the healthcare sector has been particularly slow to take advantage of the transformative power of the data already locked inside patient records. When it has become possible – and easier – to predict a potential suicide attempt from an individual's social media feeds than from their clinical notes, even though the latter are likely to contain far more clues of what is about to occur, then we are clearly missing a trick. Healthcare records can be incomplete, of poor quality and fragmented, but the biggest issue of all is actually an act of omission: the data is not used to its full potential – not even close. Some data from an individual's record might be used to help treat that individual. Patient data from multiple records may be combined to perform a variety of population-level analyses – and this is an area likely to see a renaissance in the coming years – but for a patient's data to be combined routinely with other patient data to support the care of another individual, in a day-to-day operational environment, is almost unheard of.

Centennials (Generation Z) have emerged into a world where a book recommendation that meets all their needs (subject matter, taste, ratings, likely enjoyment, number of pages, etc) can be obtained in seconds online. It was not so long ago that bestseller lists and often flaky, personal recommendations from friends returning from a recent beach holiday were all that was available. Amazon has democratised book recommendations on a global scale and in only two decades. Those same centennials must wonder why, when given a choice of treatment options for a particular condition, they are not able to do the same thing: anonymously examine the aggregated options chosen by previous patients and the outcomes they achieved in order to inform their decision making. After all, in most healthcare settings, the data is all there, sitting on the same system their data has just been entered into. Patients just can't access it.

This book is primarily about that patient data: how it could be used better, not only to improve patient outcomes but also to improve the systems and processes that produce those outcomes. Placing patients at the centre of their own care will ultimately prove vital in this. Patient-centred care has been an aspiration for many years but it has never really been reflected in the design of healthcare IT systems. Clinicians too have often been underserved by IT; they are rarely involved in system specification to an adequate level and applications consequently don't reflect the reality of day-to-day workflows, or are unable to adapt flexibly when those workflows change.

This book is also about the next generation of patient record systems – the repositories of all this data – and the need for those systems to address each of these challenges.

Six themes are identified and explored:

1. **Outcomes:** Why outcomes are sometimes confused with inputs to the detriment of patient care and why measuring true outcomes is essential to improving population health in its widest sense.
2. **Care pathways:** Why, in a data-driven healthcare system, it pays to standardise in order to provide effective personalised care.

3. **Decision support:** Why it is necessary to invest as much in getting information out of our systems as we do getting data in.
4. **Workflow:** How optimising processes for clinicians allows them to spend more time on patient care and less time on administrative tasks.
5. **Interoperability:** Why it is essential to get systems to talk to each other to optimise patient care and avoid system mediocrity.
6. **Patient first:** What is meant by patient-centred care and in what ways should this be reflected in the design of digital health records.

There is no particular order of importance to these themes and in real-world scenarios elements of each will often need to be referenced and combined. From the perspective of an application developer, this means that any given project to design, say, a new module should be tested against the list to see how many of the themes are addressed. Those projects that tick the most boxes are likely to produce the most benefits.

First and foremost, the primary purpose of my writing this book is to encourage all of us working in the healthcare community to use the data and the emerging technology to promote the idea of data-driven healthcare as succinctly represented in the formula below:

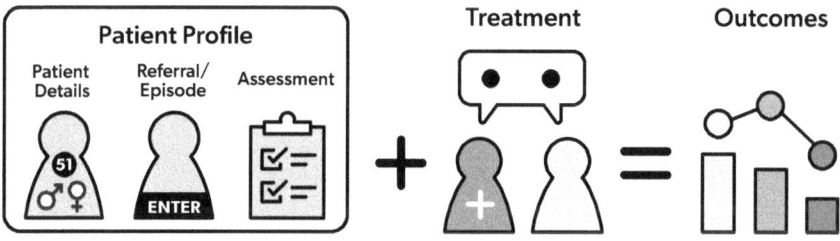

Today, every patient who embarks on a healthcare journey will achieve some kind of outcome that we can measure. By building an appropriate profile of each patient, recording their healthcare journey systematically and then capturing their resulting outcomes, we can build up a database of interventions that is both standardised for all patients while also being personalised for each individual. Then the magic happens, because we can subsequently use all these historic records to build up a picture of what works and what doesn't for different types of patient and in real time predict outcomes for the patient in front of us now and those arriving tomorrow. As more and more patient journeys are added, the potential to help future patients becomes greater and greater.

The time for data-driven healthcare has finally arrived. The vision for a new approach to patient management presented in these pages is not far reaching; technology is moving so fast that new possibilities are emerging all the time. Rather it is an attempt to win over hearts and minds and garner support for a philosophy that puts patient data very much into the mix in optimising care, and to set an agenda for the next generation of software that builds on and advances where the industry is today. I also recognised that this vision does not exist in a technological vacuum even in the current environment. Consequently, the opening chapters outline the key emerging innovations and challenges that look set to drive the healthcare agenda and technology landscape over the coming years. I then go on to examine the role of data and data systems in that landscape, explore the emerging themes summarised above together with their role in data-driven healthcare and the challenges we will need to overcome in getting there.

2 The challenge for healthcare

Healthcare systems across the world are under pressure. Demand is outstripping supply at an ever-increasing rate. In this chapter, I examine the key factors driving this demand.

Demographics

Two macro demographic trends are challenging the healthcare system. First, populations are getting bigger. As I write, the world population stands at more than 8.2 billion. By 2050, not that far away, it is projected to be just short of 10 billion. That's 20 per cent more people on the planet in the next 25 years. Put another way, that's five more United States – all with healthcare needs.

The other significant demographic trend is that populations are growing older, particularly in developed countries. According to the UK Office for National Statistics, in 1997, one in six people was over the age of 65. By 2017, that figure had climbed to almost one in five, fuelled partly by the baby boom generation. By 2037, the over 65s will represent one in four of the population (ONS 2018). Globally, life expectancy has risen from 47 years in 1950 to 72 years in 2022 and rising (Richter 2023). That's not just more healthcare demand due to the growing number of people, but more complex and long-term needs due to the naturally associated rise in chronic conditions that come with old age – more heart disease, more cancer, more dementia. While the average life expectancy has risen to 73 years across both sexes, the average years of healthy life is only 63 (ONS 2017). This means, on average, ten years of life are spent in poor health.

Despite these overall trends for the global population as a whole, they are not universally true at regional level. Huge improvements in infant mortality over the past few decades now require women in almost every country to give birth to only two children on average to maintain the population. However, actual fertility rates, which have been falling steadily since 1950, still vary widely. Around 100 nations are not producing enough children to keep their population level, while in a similar number of countries the opposite is true and high birth rates are driving population increases. Not surprisingly, perhaps, the developing nations continue to deliver the higher birth rates while many developed nations are now listed among those with a birth rate of less than two per adult pair. In a generation, these trends will create more baby booms and busts for those countries, with consequences for both their economies and healthcare systems.

Disease burden

Inevitably, as the global population increases and grows older, the diseases associated with old age become more prevalent. Mortality is now a complex thing to untangle as older adults often tend to die with a range of deteriorating conditions (known as co-morbidities in health-speak), any of which would have ultimately resulted in death. But even the causes of early death have shifted. In the first half of the 20th century, lower respiratory infections and diarrheal diseases were the primary causes of death globally; for some decades now they have been replaced by ischaemic heart disease and stroke. In general, early deaths from enteric and respiratory infections have fallen, together with infant mortality due to neonatal and congenital disorders. Meanwhile, progress in reducing mortality from non-communicable diseases, such as cardiovascular disease and cancers, has stalled or reversed. Furthermore, mortality from diseases and disorders linked to antibiotic resistance has been an unintended consequence of greater access to healthcare globally.

The most marked trends have arisen not in changes in mortality, but in the incidence of chronic conditions. The burden of disability is concentrated in people of working age and is primarily composed of musculoskeletal disorders, non-communicable conditions such as cancers, cardiovascular and pulmonary diseases, and metabolic conditions such as diabetes and chronic kidney disease. Mental illness, including neurological disorders, has also been on the rise. Collectively, the marked downward trend in the burden of communicable disease (Covid aside) has been more than offset by a rapid rise in non-communicable conditions. Only a minority of disability today is caused by communicable diseases and this is primarily the burden of developing nations. In the developed world, the two leading causes of disability have remained lower back pain and headache, while depression and diabetes have both seen dramatic rises.

Perhaps the most telling shift in the global disease burden has not been in the diseases themselves but in the risk factors associated with those diseases. Twenty-five years ago, the highest risk factors contributing to early death were related to gestational metrics (ie measurements used to assess the age and development of a foetus during pregnancy) and child nutrition. Today, they are high blood pressure, high blood sugar and smoking.

These trends are set to continue. Twenty years from now, the top ten causes of early death globally are expected to contain only one category of communicable disease (lower respiratory infections) compared with six today. Heart disease and stroke will maintain the top two places but the rest of the list will be dominated by rising chronic conditions, including chronic obstructive pulmonary disease (COPD), kidney disease, diabetes, Alzheimer's disease and lung cancer.

Financial pressures

Meeting the global annual healthcare needs of 8.2 billion people is now estimated to cost more than US$10 trillion, averaging over US$1,200 for every person alive. Low-income countries spend less than US$50 per person per year, while high-income countries spend around US$4,000 per person. Spending on healthcare overall represents just over 10 per cent of global GDP. All of the trends highlighted in this chapter are driving healthcare costs ever skyward. By 2030, the global spend is projected to rise to US$15 trillion with a world population reaching 8.5 billion by the end of the year, an increase of 45 per cent in the average cost per person in just five years (RBC Capital Markets 2025).

There are clearly wide-ranging variations in healthcare spending from country to country and this is expected to continue. Over the next few years, this spending will be driven by the common headwinds of ageing and growing populations but in many countries by the additional pressures of clinical and technology advances and rising labour costs. Healthcare markets in developing nations in particular are expected to see rapid expansion.

The trend toward universal healthcare is also expected to accelerate with more governments allocating a greater proportion of their spending budgets toward their public healthcare systems. Yet despite continual funding increases in many countries, expenditure on public health systems is failing to counter a range of persistent challenges. These include accessibility, caused by an imbalanced distribution of resources and urban/rural and other geopolitical divides; affordability, for people on low incomes or without adequate insurance; awareness of vaccination benefits, health risks and lifestyle diseases; a lack of clinical and technical skills; and inadequate or non-existent infrastructure.

Public healthcare spending pressures are particularly prevalent in Australia and the UK. In England, at the nadir of the global financial crisis in 2011, just 5 per cent of National Health Service (NHS) trusts breached their annual spending budgets (Burton et al 2021). Five years later, two thirds of trusts were in deficit as austerity took its toll (King's Fund 2022). Despite a subsequent injection of funds into the system, as we entered 2025, almost all of the 42 integrated care boards were spending more than their budgets, driven mainly by deficits in their local trusts. Analysis shows that hospital spending continues to be the largest contributory factor, despite a range of initiatives to move care into the community where services have seen relatively little investment. At the same time, patients are finding it increasingly difficult to obtain appointments with their general practitioner. One of the highest growth rates in public health care spending has been seen in Australia, which saw a 72 per cent increase between 2012 and 2022 (AIHW 2024). The Australian federal government has reacted by pressuring the newly formed primary health networks (PHNs) to drive innovation that delivers sustainable cost controls.

In a global environment where inexorable demand for healthcare is outstripping available resources, there are few options to bridge the gap. But technology is one of them. Despite the urgency of all the challenges, and a usable internet that is now 25 years old, the world has only just begun to explore the potential for digital to revolutionise the healthcare system. Significant investments will need to be made to unleash the healing power of the data but the potential returns over the coming years could be enormous.

Better diagnostics

History has not always reflected the true burden of disease. Many people today suffer from diseases that have only recently been categorised. Many more have died without their cause of death having been reliably diagnosed. This makes the process of monitoring disease trends very difficult. Is the burden of any particular disease genuinely higher today or is it simply that detection systems have improved?

No doubt the world is getting better at diagnosis. Indeed, new tests and techniques are increasing exponentially, but this will only add to the pressures on the healthcare system: the more diagnostics are performed, the more resulting treatments are needed. But at least they will be the right treatments.

Briefly, here are the current technology trends in available clinical diagnostics:

- ❖ **Genomics:** Genetic sequencing has seen dramatic improvements in both accuracy and affordability over the past few years. The pervasiveness of sequencing platforms, and platforms for library preparation, are now making

the technology more widely available, opening the door to widespread personalisation of test results.
- ❖ **Automation:** The rise of genetic testing has been fuelled by the increased availability of automation technologies, which bring down the cost while driving higher throughputs and greater flexibility. As a result, genotyping is now available to consumers. Automated storage and retrieval systems, coupled with robotics, provide even greater scope for personalised diagnostic profiling, which heralds a new era in truly patient-centric medicine.
- ❖ **Point of care:** Diagnostic delivery is being greatly impacted by the emergence of new point-of-care technologies (POCT), which provide actionable information at the site of care to allow rapid clinical decision making. Applications include continuous monitoring or spot testing, and these can be delivered through a range of technologies, including smartphones, wearables, non-invasive devices, paper-based diagnostics, nanopore-based devices and digital microfluidics (both enabling molecular-level scanning).
- ❖ **Complexity:** More tests, more samples, more experimental variations, more genomics – all these factors have resulted in the world of clinical diagnostics becoming more complex and increasingly a data problem. Advances in analytics have improved the understanding of genomics in particular, by revealing hidden patterns, unknown correlations and other insights. Cloud computing is making it easier to collaborate, share and analyse large datasets in real time. Machine-learning algorithms will reveal even more insights and use them to make predictions.

I will return to these in the following chapters. But as new diagnostic technologies become increasingly ubiquitous and consumer based, the problems they find and the treatments they point to will grow in number, further fuelling demand for those interventions.

New interventions

As technology expands the diagnostic landscape, so too the range of interventions on offer continues to grow. New treatments that are shown not to improve outcomes over traditional interventions will fail to gain traction (unless they are significantly cheaper) and disappear into obscurity, so inevitably the best treatments available are the latest ones. Given the regulatory environment in which they are developed – and the vast and increasing number of hurdles required to be overcome before adoption – they also tend to be the most expensive.

Of course, many of these new interventions are drugs for which the journey to market requires deep pockets and bucketfuls of patience. Often, in order to recoup their investment, companies set prices that the healthcare system cannot afford, or where impossible choices have to be made in the allocation of spending budgets. Different healthcare commissioners may make different choices, spawning a postcode lottery. Non-pharmaceutical interventions (ie any physical or psychological treatment not requiring drugs) are increasingly subject to similar regimes, further inflating the ethical dilemmas.

Technologically driven improvements in interventions do not necessarily have to follow this pattern and, in the battle to close the gap between ever-increasing demand and constrained budgets, new technological advances perhaps offer the only light at the end of the tunnel. In the following chapters, I sweep through the current technological landscape and scan the horizon for the knights in shining armour that may yet save the day.

3 Emerging technology trends

While this book is focused on data-driven healthcare, and particularly on the next generation of patient care record systems, it is important to recognise that advances in digital and data technology are not being undertaken in a vacuum. The landscape of technological developments in medicine and healthcare is expanding rapidly, and some important trends are already beginning to take root. This chapter provides a broad overview of the landscape and will hopefully act as a useful summary of the current state of the art. However, if you wish to maintain a focus on the primary subject of this book – data-driven healthcare – feel free to skim read the subheadings or skip it altogether.

Remote patient-centric technologies and applications

In an ideal world, we wouldn't need hospitals at all. Given the choice, most patients would prefer to continue with as normal a life as possible and remain in their own homes. Hospitals can also be dangerous – particularly for sicker patients – and hospital-acquired infections are unfortunately far from unusual. With demand soaring, bed numbers at historically low levels, together with challenges discharging patients into community and social care settings, hospitals are today running at full capacity – or greater. There are therefore many reasons why we would want to invest in technologies that support the care of patients outside of hospital and fortunately this domain has expanded rapidly over the past few years.

Telehealth

Telehealth is a broad term describing a rapidly developing range of technologies that allows patients to receive medical care remotely, away from traditional healthcare facilities. Instead of waiting for face-to-face appointments with their doctor, patients access care through their digital devices, using personalised mobile apps to communicate virtually with medical professionals to receive instant diagnosis and medical advice. Telehealth is particularly relevant for patients managing chronic conditions as it provides them with consistent, convenient and cost-effective care. Today, use of remote healthcare delivery is especially prevalent in mental health services, where a growing number of online platforms are proving to be as effective as face-to-face therapy, while also offering both flexibility and easier access, and reducing the volume and impact of missed appointments.

With increasingly overstretched services, telehealth provides patients with more options to access healthcare at their own convenience. It is believed that more than half of patients prefer digitally led services and the global market for telemedicine has already exceeded $100bn per annum and is set to triple by the beginning of the next decade (BusinessWire 2025).

Remote patient monitoring

The ability to track patients' vital signs and health metrics from their homes represents one of the most significant shifts in healthcare delivery. Using connected devices such as smart watches, blood pressure monitors and glucose sensors, doctors can now receive real-time health data without requiring patients to visit medical facilities.

This continuous monitoring creates a more complete picture of health than occasional clinic visits, allowing for earlier intervention when problems arise. For those with chronic conditions such as heart disease or diabetes, remote monitoring has already been shown to reduce hospital readmissions and emergency visits. The technology is particularly valuable for elderly patients or those in rural areas, for whom travel to medical appointments presents significant challenges. As these systems become more sophisticated, they'll likely incorporate AI to identify concerning patterns before they become medical emergencies, alerting healthcare providers to check in with patients. The result will be a move away from reactive care toward preventative intervention, potentially saving countless lives while reducing the overall burden on healthcare systems.

Remote therapeutic monitoring

Remote therapeutic monitoring systems track patients' progress during rehabilitation and other therapy programmes, using sensors and mobile applications to collect data on exercise adherence, functional improvements and symptom changes between clinical visits. Unlike general remote monitoring, these systems focus specifically on measuring therapeutic outcomes and adherence to prescribed treatment plans.

For physiotherapy patients recovering from surgery or injury, wearable sensors can measure range of motion, exercise form and progress on specific functional goals, providing therapists with objective data to guide treatment adjustments. In speech therapy, voice analysis applications can track improvements in articulation or fluency, while occupational therapy patients might use smart utensils or other instrumented tools that measure fine motor control improvements. The technology creates a continuous record of patient progress rather than relying solely on periodic in-clinic assessments, allowing earlier intervention when recovery plateaus or regresses. For providers, these systems help prioritise which patients need additional attention or modified treatment plans. Recently, medical insurance policies have specifically supported remote therapeutic monitoring, resulting in accelerated adoption across rehabilitation specialties. Again, the approach has shown to be particularly valuable for rural patients who might otherwise travel long distances for brief therapy sessions, and for monitoring compliance with home exercise programmes, which are traditionally a major challenge in rehabilitation medicine.

By extending therapeutic oversight beyond clinic walls, these technologies are transforming rehabilitation from periodic professional interactions to continuous guided recovery supported by granular, objective data.

Wearables

In healthcare, wearable technology primarily refers to electronic devices such as smart watches, which are designed to collect users' personal health and exercise data. In particular, wearable fitness technology is now mainstream. According to research, between around 60 and 80 per cent of consumers are willing to wear fitness monitoring devices (Jia et al 2018). Consequently, the use of wearables is currently tripling every four years and shows no sign of slowing down (Cartan Capital 2023).

Today, wearables take a number of forms:

- **Wearable fitness trackers:** These represent the simplest forms of wearable technology in the form of wristbands equipped with sensors that track the user's physical activity and heart rate, capturing and analysing the data using smartphone apps.
- **Smart health watches:** These are gradually transforming into clinically viable healthcare devices, able to monitor an increasing range of metrics, such as heart rhythms (to alert patients with atrial fibrillation), sleep patterns and movement (used for a number of mental health conditions and Parkinson's sufferers).
- **Wearable ECG monitors:** Taking smartwatches to another level, wearable ECGs produce more detailed electrocardiograms and can alert doctors should a problem be detected.
- **Wearable blood pressure monitors:** These devices offer all the features of a smart watch and heart monitor but with the addition of an oscillometric blood pressure monitor.
- **Biosensors:** Radically different from wrist trackers and smart watches, biosensors have now arrived in the form of

self-adhesive patches that will in time collect an increasing range of biometric data.

In high-risk groups, the adoption of wearable technology has been shown to significantly reduce preventable cardiac or respiratory arrest and results like this are exciting both healthcare providers and insurers alike (Odeh et al 2024). Wearable technology encourages users to engage with their health and incentivises behaviour that reduces hospital visits and readmissions due to poorly managed lifestyles.

Continuous glucose monitoring systems

Continuous glucose monitoring systems, in particular, have transformed diabetes management by providing real-time blood sugar readings without the finger pricks previously required for testing. These wearable devices use tiny sensors inserted just under the skin to measure glucose levels in interstitial fluid, transmitting readings to smartphones or dedicated receivers every few minutes.

For diabetes patients, this constant stream of data reveals patterns and trends invisible to traditional testing methods, showing how meals, exercise, medications and stress affect blood sugar throughout the day and night. Advanced systems now include predictive alerts that warn users of potential highs or lows before they happen, allowing preventative action rather than reactive treatment. Integration with insulin pumps has created 'closed-loop' artificial pancreas systems that automatically adjust insulin delivery based on glucose readings, dramatically improving blood sugar control. The technology has extended beyond type 1 diabetes to help those with type 2 diabetes optimise their treatment plans, and even to non-diabetic populations interested in metabolic health. Recent developments include smaller, more accurate sensors with longer wearing times and systems designed specifically for paediatric patients. By providing unprecedented visibility into glucose patterns, these devices have improved treatment adherence, reduced emergency hospitalisations and given millions of diabetes patients greater control over their condition.

Wireless sensors

Extending the revolution in wearable technology further will no doubt involve the development of wireless body area networks (WBANs), a specialised type of wireless sensor network (WSN) dedicated to monitoring vital healthcare metrics unobtrusively while patients continue with their lives. WBANs take data from a variety of sensors, both wearable and internal, to build a more holistic and continuous picture of a patient's state of health, broadening the abilities of wearables by including metrics on chemical imbalances in the body in addition to monitoring cardiac function, fitness and temperature.

Some of these new wireless sensors are now bioresorbable – electronic devices that can be placed in the body and dissolve when they are no longer needed – reducing the need for additional surgery. These will be especially useful in monitoring vital metrics in the brain.

WBANs are most likely to be deployed not on individual patients but on whole groups or even populations. Data transmitted onto the wireless network could be captured at a central point and monitored by a dedicated team operating out of a control centre linked to GPs, hospitals and emergency services.

Advanced wound care technologies

Smart bandages and advanced dressings have revolutionised wound treatment by incorporating sensors, medication delivery systems and healing stimulation technologies directly into wound coverings. These sophisticated dressings monitor healing progress in real time while actively intervening to improve outcomes.

For patients with chronic wounds such as diabetic ulcers or pressure sores, sensor-equipped bandages can detect early signs of infection by measuring pH changes, temperature fluctuations or specific bacterial markers before symptoms become visible. Some advanced dressings incorporate electrical stimulation or ultrasound technologies that accelerate tissue repair by increasing local blood flow and cellular activity. Others contain embedded medication reservoirs that release antimicrobials or growth factors in response to specific biological triggers detected in the wound environment. Data from these smart bandages can be transmitted wirelessly to healthcare providers, enabling remote monitoring without removing dressings – a process that often disrupts healing and increases infection risk. For the millions of patients with chronic wounds, particularly elderly individuals and those with diabetes, these technologies can prevent complications that might otherwise lead to hospitalisation or amputation. While more expensive than traditional dressings, their ability to detect complications early and accelerate healing ultimately reduces overall treatment costs while significantly improving patient quality of life and clinical outcomes.

Ingestible sensors

Ingestible sensor technology has moved from concept to clinical reality with systems that can verify medication ingestion and collect internal health data through tiny devices swallowed with pills or as standalone capsules. About the size of a grain of sand, these sensors are activated by stomach fluids and transmit signals to external patches worn on the patient's body.

For patients with serious mental illnesses, medication adherence sensors can confirm antipsychotic ingestion, addressing a major challenge in schizophrenia and bipolar disorder management where non-adherence frequently leads to relapse and hospitalisation.

Once ingested, the sensor transmits a signal to a smartphone application, allowing patients, caregivers and clinicians to track medication patterns objectively rather than relying on self-reporting. Diagnostic ingestible sensors can measure internal body temperature, detect gastrointestinal bleeding or monitor acid levels throughout the digestive tract, providing information previously requiring invasive procedures. Advanced research versions can sample the microbiome or intestinal fluid for biomarkers as they pass through the digestive system.

The technology raises important privacy considerations, requiring careful consent processes and data protection. However, for conditions where medication adherence is critical or internal monitoring would otherwise require invasive procedures, these sensors offer a dramatically less intrusive alternative. By making the invisible visible – whether medication-taking behaviour or internal physiological processes – ingestible sensors represent one of the most innovative approaches to health monitoring currently in clinical use.

Portable diagnostic devices

Portable diagnostic devices are bringing laboratory-quality testing out of centralised facilities and into point-of-care settings, dramatically reducing waiting times for critical results. These compact systems can perform tests ranging from blood chemistry panels to infectious disease detection using minimal samples and delivering results in minutes rather than days.

For emergency departments, these devices enable rapid diagnosis of conditions such as heart attacks, sepsis or stroke, allowing treatment to begin without waiting for results to be returned from a central laboratory. In primary care practices, clinicians can make immediate treatment decisions during patient visits rather than following up days later. The technology has shown to be particularly valuable in rural and low-resource settings where traditional laboratory access is limited, enabling sophisticated diagnostics in locations previously served only by basic testing.

Recent advances include smartphone-connected devices that turn mobile phones into diagnostic platforms for conditions ranging from urinary tract infections to Covid-19, with results that approach laboratory accuracy. Many systems are designed for use by non-specialists, widening access to diagnostic capabilities beyond traditional medical settings. While questions remain about quality control and standardisation across different platforms, regulatory agencies have established frameworks for validating these technologies.

By bringing sophisticated testing capabilities directly to patient care settings, portable diagnostics are fundamentally changing how and where crucial medical decisions are made, potentially saving countless lives through faster intervention.

Digital healthcare programmes

This is the age of digital, so it is no surprise that, like many other aspects of our lives, banking or shopping for example, healthcare can also be delivered digitally in certain circumstances. A digital health programme is a structured initiative that leverages technology to improve health outcomes, healthcare delivery and health education. These programmes typically incorporate digital tools such as the wearable devices and telemedicine platforms described above, but augment these with mobile applications and online resources to enhance patient monitoring, facilitate remote care, provide personalised health information and promote positive behaviour changes.

Digital health programmes can address various health needs, from chronic disease management to preventive care, mental health support and wellness promotion, while often reducing barriers to healthcare access and potentially lowering overall healthcare costs.

Digital therapy

Unlike traditional healthcare apps that simply track health data, digital therapeutics are software-based interventions that prevent, manage or treat medical disorders. Unlike wellness apps, these products undergo clinical trials like conventional medications and can be prescribed by doctors, representing a fundamentally new treatment category.

Digital therapeutics already exist for conditions including anxiety and depression, substance abuse, chronic insomnia and ADHD, delivering cognitive behavioural therapy and other evidence-based interventions through smartphones and tablets. They typically include interactive modules, progress tracking and personalised feedback based on user responses and engagement patterns. For patients with chronic conditions, whether physical or mental, these tools provide accessible and consistent support between medical appointments, helping them make daily decisions that improve their health.

The appeal extends beyond convenience. Digital therapeutics can adapt to individual needs, becoming more personalised as they gather data on a user's responses and progress. They are particularly promising for behavioural health conditions, where access to qualified therapists remains limited in many regions or out of hours.

As regulatory frameworks evolve to accommodate this new treatment category, we will likely see digital therapeutics becoming standard components of care plans, working alongside traditional medications and therapies to improve outcomes across a wide range of (mainly chronic) conditions, from diabetes management to depression treatment.

Virtual and augmented reality therapy

Virtual reality (VR) and augmented reality (AR) technologies are transforming physical rehabilitation and mental health treatment by creating immersive therapeutic environments.

For physiotherapy patients, VR can gamify recovery exercises, increasing engagement and adherence to treatment plans. The technology can also distract from pain during procedures or recovery, in some cases reducing the need for medication.

In mental health, VR exposure therapy helps patients confront phobias and anxiety triggers in controlled environments, where therapists can adjust the intensity of experiences based on a patient's progress. For PTSD sufferers, these tools provide safe ways to process trauma without the risks of real-world exposure. As the technology becomes more accessible and affordable, it will no doubt become integrated into home treatment plans, expanding access to specialised therapy regardless of location. The next generation of these systems will likely incorporate biofeedback, allowing therapists to monitor physiological responses during sessions and tailor treatments accordingly.

This immersive approach to therapy represents a fundamental shift in how we approach both physical and psychological healing, potentially making treatments more effective and accessible for millions of patients worldwide.

Digital mental health interventions

Building on the above, mental health treatments specifically have already become a significant beneficiary. Mental health services face unprecedented demand amid a global shortage of providers, leaving many patients without access to timely care. Digital interventions – including the aforementioned smartphone-based therapy apps, virtual reality exposure treatments and AI chatbots – are proving invaluable in helping to bridge this gap by making evidence-based approaches available regardless of location or provider accessibility.

These technologies not only offer complete accessibility, allowing patients to receive support outside traditional office hours and in the privacy of their own homes, but also help combat the stigma that prevents many from seeking help. For mild to moderate psychological conditions, digital interventions have shown effectiveness comparable to in-person therapy in multiple clinical trials, though they're generally positioned as supplements rather than replacements for human providers in more severe cases.

The continuous nature of digital support also addresses a fundamental limitation of traditional therapy. Instead of weekly sessions, patients can receive guidance during actual moments of distress or when practising new coping skills. As artificial intelligence improves, these systems will likely become more responsive to individual needs, recognising emotional states from text patterns, voice characteristics or even facial expressions captured by smartphone cameras.

While digital approaches won't replace human connection in mental healthcare, they represent a promising way to extend limited resources and provide consistent support between traditional sessions, potentially transforming how we address the growing global burden of mental health conditions.

Digital therapeutics for addiction treatment

Digital addiction treatments have also emerged as evidence-based interventions for substance use disorders, combining cognitive behavioural therapy techniques with modern engagement strategies in smartphone applications. These programmes deliver structured therapeutic content, coping skills training and motivational exercises accessible any time patients face cravings or triggers.

For people struggling with addiction, particularly those in areas with limited treatment resources, these applications again provide consistent support between formal therapy sessions or as standalone interventions for those unable to access traditional programmes. Many incorporate features such as progress tracking, personalised feedback and community support through moderated discussion forums where users can safely share experiences.

Some advanced systems include biometric monitoring through smartphone sensors or connected devices, detecting stress patterns that might precede relapse and providing intervention at critical moments. Several applications have undergone rigorous clinical trials demonstrating effectiveness comparable to certain in-person interventions, leading to regulatory approval and, increasingly, insurance coverage. The technology proved particularly valuable during the Covid-19 pandemic, when in-person treatment access was limited, and once again for patients in rural areas who might otherwise travel hours to reach specialised addiction services.

While not replacing human connection entirely, these digital tools extend the reach of evidence-based addiction treatments to populations historically underserved by traditional recovery resources (eg ethnic minorities, hard-to-reach groups or simply those living in areas with different spending priorities), potentially addressing a critical gap in substance use treatment.

Diagnostic systems

As I alluded to in the previous chapter, digital technologies have fundamentally transformed diagnostic services, revolutionising how healthcare providers detect, analyse and monitor medical conditions. Through innovations such as artificial intelligence algorithms, advanced imaging techniques, remote monitoring devices and digitised laboratory systems, clinicians can now achieve greater diagnostic accuracy, speed and accessibility than ever before. These technologies enable earlier disease detection, more precise identification of subtle abnormalities and the ability to process vast amounts of patient data to support clinical decision making. New technologies have also facilitated the migration of diagnostic facilities from hospitals into community-based geographical settings. I have already described how digital diagnostic tools have expanded healthcare reach through telehealth platforms, allowing for remote consultations and evaluations, while integrated electronic health records ensure diagnostic information flows seamlessly across the healthcare continuum, ultimately improving patient outcomes and treatment efficiency.

In this section, I will briefly look at some specific diagnostic technologies that have emerged in recent years, both improving diagnostic accuracy and, by making internal examinations dramatically less invasive, enhancing the patient experience.

Capsule endoscopy

Capsule endoscopy has transformed gastrointestinal diagnostics by replacing traditional invasive endoscopic procedures with a swallowable camera pill. About the size of a vitamin supplement, these capsules contain miniature cameras, lights, batteries and wireless transmitters that capture thousands of images as they travel naturally through the digestive tract over eight to 12 hours.

This technology has proven particularly valuable for examining the small intestine, previously difficult to visualise with conventional endoscopy or colonoscopy. Patients simply swallow the capsule in their doctor's office and wear a small recording device on their belt that receives and stores images for later review. The procedure allows people to continue normal daily activities during the examination, eliminating the sedation, discomfort and recovery time associated with traditional scopes. Gastroenterologists use capsule endoscopy to diagnose conditions including obscure gastrointestinal bleeding, Crohn's disease, small bowel tumours and celiac disease with minimal patient discomfort.

Recent advances include capsules with multiple cameras for 360-degree views, improved battery life and AI-assisted image analysis to help doctors identify abnormalities more accurately. Next-generation capsules under development will add capabilities for tissue sampling and even delivering treatments directly to affected areas.

Liquid biopsies

Liquid biopsies detect circulating tumour DNA in blood samples, offering a minimally invasive alternative to surgical tissue biopsies for cancer diagnosis, monitoring and treatment selection. These blood tests can identify genetic mutations and other cancer markers released into the bloodstream by tumour cells throughout the body.

For cancer patients, the technology eliminates the pain, complications and recovery time associated with traditional tissue biopsies, while allowing for more frequent monitoring of treatment response. Liquid biopsies can detect cancer recurrence months before it becomes visible on imaging studies, enabling earlier intervention when treatments are most effective. The technology has proven particularly valuable for cancers such as lung cancer, where traditional biopsies carry significant risks, and for monitoring cancers that may develop resistance to targeted therapies.

Several liquid biopsy tests have received regulatory approval and entered clinical practice, particularly for selecting patients who might benefit from specific targeted therapies based on their cancer's genetic profile. The field is advancing rapidly, with newer tests capable of detecting more genetic alterations with greater sensitivity and specificity than earlier versions. While not yet replacing traditional biopsies in all contexts, liquid biopsies are increasingly complementing conventional methods in oncology practice.

By providing crucial genetic information through a simple blood sample, this technology is transforming how oncologists monitor and treat cancer.

Voice-based disease detection

Voice analysis technologies use AI to identify subtle vocal biomarkers associated with various health conditions, potentially enabling earlier diagnosis through simple speaking tasks. These systems analyse numerous acoustic features in speech that humans cannot perceive, detecting patterns associated with conditions ranging from Parkinson's disease to depression.

For neurological disorders – like Parkinson's – the technology can identify subtle speech changes months or even years before traditional diagnostic methods would detect the condition, potentially allowing earlier intervention. Similar applications are showing promise for respiratory conditions, with distinctive speech patterns emerging in patients with conditions like chronic obstructive pulmonary disease (COPD), even before breathing difficulties become apparent. Mental health applications include identifying vocal patterns associated with depression, anxiety and even suicide risk, potentially providing objective measurements in a field historically reliant on subjective assessments.

The technology is particularly appealing because voice samples can be collected remotely using ordinary smartphones, making screening possible without clinic visits. Some vocal biomarker algorithms are already beginning to receive regulatory clearance as adjunctive diagnostic tools (eg for Covid-19 in the UK and amyotrophic lateral sclerosis, ALS, in the US), though they are not yet fully approved or standard in clinical practice. However, the non-invasive nature of the technology and its potential for remote deployment make it one of the most accessible emerging diagnostic approaches, potentially enabling widespread, low-cost screening for conditions where early detection significantly improves outcomes.

Genomics

Although expectations of a brave new clinical world associated with an increased focus on DNA have been around since the 1960s, it took until 2003 for the entire human genome – all the hereditary information encoded in DNA – to be mapped. The original project cost almost $3 billion spent over 13 years. By 2006, the cost of sequencing an individual genome had fallen to $300,000 (Meskó 2017). Today a plethora of companies offer people the opportunity to map their entire genome for $1,000 or less, with the results provided in more detail and in a matter of hours. A test for a single gene now costs less than $150.

Genomics – the combination of genetics and medicine – has heralded a wave of predictive medicine, which aims to assess a person's risk of succumbing to a disease that may have killed, or curtailed the life of, their ancestors. Today, these tests are routinely used for women with a family history of breast cancer – or men whose fathers had prostate cancer – yet while the accuracy of these predictions has improved, they are not yet good enough, in any area, to determine definitively whether someone will ultimately be a victim or not. As a result, predictive medicine does have a dark side, which can result in people developing anxiety-based mental health conditions or having ultimately unnecessary preventative procedures, with all the inherent risks that any form of surgery or drug regimen involves.

Personalised medicine

Medical interventions do not affect all patients the same way. People are unique and individual responses to new medications and implants, as key examples, will be equally varied. Until today, working out which drug will suit which patient best has been mostly trial and error.

The dramatic reduction in the cost of genome sequencing has opened the door to truly personalised medicine, where treatments are tailored to a patient's unique genetic make-up. From a simple blood sample or cheek swab, doctors can now identify genetic variants that affect how patients will respond to medications, allowing for more precise dosing and reducing adverse reactions.

In cancer care, genomic testing is already helping oncologists select treatments targeted to specific tumour mutations, improving outcomes while minimising unnecessary side effects. As the understanding of genetic influences on disease progresses, it is likely that there will be customised prevention plans based on individual risk factors, potentially heading off diseases before they develop.

While genetic-based technologies raise important privacy concerns that must be addressed, the potential of a genomic approach to medicine to transform patient outcomes makes it one of the most promising healthcare innovations on the horizon, particularly for complex conditions that have historically been difficult to treat effectively.

Pharmacogenomics

Pharmacogenomics (the study of how genes affect drug responses) is a specific branch of personalised medicine and is destined to become standard practice, dramatically reducing the trial-and-error approach to medication selection that frustrates both doctors and patients today. By analysing a patient's genetic profile to predict how they will respond to specific medications, pharmacogenomic testing – using only a simple blood sample or cheek swab – allows doctors to select the most effective drugs and dosages based on individual genetic markers.

For patients, this technology can prevent adverse drug reactions that hospitalise millions annually. The testing is particularly valuable for psychiatric medications, cancer treatments and pain management – areas where response variability between patients has traditionally been high. Growing evidence shows that evolving from a one-size-fits-all approach to pharmacogenomic-guided prescribing reduces side effects, improves treatment adherence and produces better outcomes across multiple specialties.

While initially limited to specialised settings, costs have decreased significantly, making the technology increasingly accessible in routine care. Major health systems have begun implementing pharmacogenomic testing into their electronic health records, flagging potential genetic incompatibilities when physicians order certain medications. Unlike most genetic tests that provide one-time results, pharmacogenomic findings remain relevant throughout a patient's life, informing medication decisions across different conditions and specialties. By eliminating much of the guesswork traditionally involved in prescribing, this technology represents a fundamental shift toward truly personalised medicine in everyday clinical practice.

Precision cancer vaccines

Personalised cancer vaccines represent one of the most promising recent advances in oncology, using the genetic profile of a patient's specific tumour to create customised immunotherapies. Unlike traditional vaccines that prevent disease, these treatments stimulate the immune system to recognise and attack cancer cells already present in the body.

The process begins with genetic sequencing of a patient's tumour to identify mutations creating proteins not found in healthy cells. Scientists then design a vaccine containing fragments of these mutated proteins, training the patient's immune system to recognise them as foreign and mount an attack specifically targeting cancer cells while sparing normal tissue. Early clinical trials have shown promising results across multiple cancer types, particularly when combined with other immunotherapy approaches. For patients with cancers that have historically responded poorly to standard treatments (eg melanoma, pancreatic, kidney, head and neck, and bowel cancers), these personalised vaccines offer a precisely targeted alternative with potentially fewer side effects than traditional chemotherapy. The technology has advanced rapidly from theoretical concept to clinical reality, with several pharmaceutical companies and research institutions conducting late-stage trials for various cancer types (see Mount Sinai 2025, for example). While manufacturing these individualised treatments remains complex and expensive, production processes are becoming more streamlined.

Epigenetics

Genes play an important role in determining the risk of certain diseases or the likely response that will be achieved by specific drugs. But at best they provide an incomplete picture. It is now clear that people with the same genes (eg identical twins) do not manifest the same diseases or respond to drug regimens the same way. This is down to their epigenetic profile, which derives from a different part of the cell and determines how genes are expressed. While genes are mainly fixed, which is why we can use them to trace ancestry, epigenetic profiles are also inherited but can change over time, depending on environmental factors such as life traumas, diet or disease. These changes can then be passed down to future generations.

Epigenetics has profound implications for both predictive and personalised medicine as it is now clear that examining an individual's genome alone does not provide a full enough picture to ever be precise enough with recommended interventions. Indeed, studying a person's epigenetic trends gives much greater insight into where their health is heading than a simple genetic screen. It is also the reason why the 'one size fits all' approach adopted in popular medicine has proved to be at best misleading and occasionally completely misguided.

The field of epigenetics is advancing faster than ever with new technologies and breakthroughs in understanding occurring on an almost daily basis. Soon, a simple saliva test will enable anyone to take personal steps to avoid their largest risk factors associated with age-related conditions such as heart disease and cancer.

Gene editing

Gene editing holds enormous potential in the prevention and treatment of disease. Today, gene editing is really all about CRISPR, which stands for clustered regularly interspaced short palindromic repeats, and refers to distinctive DNA sequences originally discovered in bacteria. The term now commonly refers to CRISPR-Cas9, a revolutionary gene-editing technology that functions like molecular scissors, allowing scientists to precisely cut and edit DNA at specific locations. The CRISPR-Cas9 system, specifically, has generated a lot of excitement because it is faster, more accurate, more efficient and cheaper than alternative methods. And while other gene editing techniques have been invented, CRISPR-Cas9 is unique in that it is based on a natural gene editing process.

Today, CRISPR is transforming medical research and treatment development across multiple fields. In agriculture, scientists are creating crops with enhanced nutritional profiles and resistance to disease and drought. In the laboratory, researchers use CRISPR to develop animal models of human diseases, helping understand conditions from cancer to Alzheimer's.

The most promising applications are in human medicine, where clinical trials are underway for CRISPR-based treatments for blood disorders such as haemophilia, sickle cell disease and beta-thalassemia and similar treatments for cystic fibrosis are being explored (Henderson 2024). These approaches remove patients' cells, edit the genetic mutation causing disease and return the corrected cells to the patient. Early results show remarkable success, with some patients effectively cured of conditions that previously required lifelong management.

In the coming years, CRISPR technology will likely become more precise with fewer errors. Next-generation CRISPR systems such as base editing and prime editing already show improved accuracy, enabling more subtle changes to individual DNA letters rather than cutting the DNA strand entirely.

The technology will likely expand to treat more common conditions such as heart disease and diabetes, potentially moving from treating existing conditions to preventing genetic diseases before symptoms develop. This progression raises profound ethical questions about where to draw boundaries, particularly regarding heritable genetic modifications that would pass to future generations.

Synthetic physiology

Synthetic physiology refers to a set of technologies that sit in the intersection of biology, engineering, and medicine – creating synthetic alternatives or enhancements to natural human biological functions. It encompasses technologies such as artificial organs, 3D bioprinting, prosthetics and exoskeletons.

3D printing

The fanfare that heralded the 3D printing era only a few years ago quickly became muted as people struggled with both the printing technology and the materials. That has all passed and 3D printing is now one of the fastest-growing technologies on the market. The medical industry has not been slow to take advantage of this new technology and 3D printing is set to play a number of important roles in the healthcare sector:

- ❖ **Prosthetics:** Precision printing allows prosthetics to be entirely bespoke to an individual patient, matching their measurements to an unprecedented level of detail, and maximising both comfort and mobility.
- ❖ **Implants:** The availability of new, safer and more durable materials paves the way for expanding the manufacture of a variety of implants using 3D printing.
- ❖ **Replicas:** Patient-specific copies of bones, organs and blood vessels can be printed to aid in the planning and execution of medical procedures.
- ❖ **Combination drugs:** 3D printers can create both enduring and soluble items. To support patients with the organisation, timing and monitoring of a complex drug regimen, 3D printing can be used to produce pills that contain multiple medications.
- ❖ **Surgical tools:** In an environment where the sterilisation of equipment is critical, the latest materials allow for the printing of one-off, throw-away instruments, as well as surgical cutting and drill guides.

Personalised 3D-printed medical devices

3D printing has revolutionised the production of medical devices by enabling rapid creation of patient-specific implants, prosthetics and surgical guides based on individual anatomy. Using digital designs created from patient imaging, these printers can produce complex three-dimensional objects layer by layer in materials ranging from plastics to metals and even biological materials.

For patients with unique anatomical needs, this technology eliminates the compromises inherent in standard, mass-produced medical devices. Surgeons now routinely use 3D-printed guides that fit precisely to a patient's bone structure during complex orthopaedic or craniofacial procedures, dramatically improving accuracy. Hearing aid manufacturers have adopted the technology to create custom-fitted devices based on digital scans of ear canals, improving comfort and performance. Perhaps most dramatically, the technology has transformed prosthetics, allowing affordable customisation that was previously prohibitively expensive. Children with growing bodies can receive updated 3D-printed prosthetics at a fraction of the cost of traditional devices, enabling more frequent replacements as they develop. Regulatory frameworks have evolved to accommodate these custom-produced medical devices, with several 3D-printed implants receiving approval for permanent placement inside the body.

By enabling precise customisation at reasonable costs, 3D printing has opened new possibilities for personalised medicine, particularly in specialties requiring anatomically specific solutions that mass manufacturing cannot efficiently provide.

3D bioprinting of tissues and organs

Unless a replacement is found, the failure of a person's vital organs will inevitably lead to death. Transplant organs have always been in short supply and many patients have died while waiting for a matching organ. Organs only become available when someone else dies and the healthcare profession is doing an ever-better job of keeping potential donors alive, exacerbating the problem. Waiting lists for heart transplants have increased by 85 per cent in ten years (Barnfield 2022). If ever the time was right for a revolution in organ availability, it is now.

Cue the dawn of the artificial organ era. Since the groundbreaking regeneration of skin cells to produce grafts for burn victims, there has been little advance in this area. That is about to change. Studies with stem cells have shown that it is possible to grow organs in the lab and titanium mechanical heart pumps are hopefully about to hit the global market.

The critical shortage of donor organs might eventually be solved through the remarkable progress in 3D bio-printing, where living cells, growth factors and biomaterials are precisely layered to create functional tissue. While complete organs are still years away from clinical use, researchers have already successfully printed blood vessels, ovaries, a thyroid gland, heart cells that actually beat and a pancreas, and are making progress on cartilage and bone replacements.

The implications for patients are profound. Waiting for donor matches could become unnecessary, and rejection risks would plummet when organs are created using a patient's own cells and therefore not triggering their immune system. Beyond transplantation, bio-printed tissues offer platforms for drug testing that more accurately reflect human biology than traditional lab models, potentially accelerating medical breakthroughs while reducing animal testing.

The technology faces significant regulatory and technical hurdles, particularly for complex organs with multiple cell types and intricate vascular networks. However, the incremental advances in printing simpler tissues are already benefiting patients, and partnerships between medical researchers and engineering experts continue to overcome limitations.

If development continues at its current pace, bio-printed organs could transform transplant medicine within the next decade, offering hope to millions worldwide awaiting life-saving surgeries.

Advanced prosthetics and exoskeletons

The integration of robotics, materials science and neural interfaces is creating a new generation of prosthetic limbs and exoskeletons that offer unprecedented functionality for people with mobility limitations. Unlike conventional prosthetics, these advanced systems can interpret electrical signals from remaining muscles or even connect directly to nerves, allowing for intuitive control that mimics natural movement.

For amputees, these developments mean prosthetics that not only look like natural limbs but function similarly, with fine motor control enabling tasks from typing to playing musical instruments. Some experimental systems even provide sensory feedback, allowing users to feel pressure or texture through their artificial limbs. For those with spinal cord injuries, powered exoskeletons are beginning to restore walking ability, providing physical independence and addressing secondary health complications associated with long-term wheelchair use. While current devices tend to be expensive and require specialised training, costs are decreasing as technologies mature and manufacturing scales up.

The next generation of these systems will likely incorporate more lightweight materials, longer-lasting power sources and improved interfaces between human and machine. As research continues, we may eventually see assistive devices that surpass natural human capabilities in certain respects – a development that would raise fascinating questions about the boundaries between rehabilitation and enhancement in medical technology.

Robots

Robots have long been used in manufacturing to improve the quality, reliability, consistency and cost-effectiveness of the manufacturing process. Healthcare, on the other hand, has been mostly seen as a system of interactions between human beings where the patient–clinician relationship is paramount to achieving excellent care. The introduction of robots into the healthcare environment has consequently been slow, but progress is being made.

Robots can play two key roles. First, they can remove repetitive and mundane tasks from busy, overstretched staff, allowing them to spend more time on the more complex or human aspects of care. As an example, robots can patrol corridors and wards, performing routine tasks such as patient observation, monitoring of vital signs and managing charts, without human intervention. Second, robots can aid in situations where mechanical precision and control are of prime importance.

Here I look at some examples, starting in the operating theatre.

Robotic surgery

Robotic surgery is now being used widely, enabling surgeons to perform complex procedures that would be otherwise highly difficult or impossible. This follows a trend which, over the past 40 years, has seen a gradual shift from open surgery to more minimally invasive approaches, which have fewer complications and a shorter recovery time. Initially this was through endoscopic and laparoscopic techniques. The use of robotic platforms for more complex procedures has increased dramatically in the past decade, and major hospital centres are seeing investments in the technology being used across multiple clinical specialties.

Robotic surgeons translate a human surgeon's hand movements into smaller, more precise actions while filtering out natural tremors, enabling complex procedures through minimal incisions. Robotic surgery is easier to learn and offers improved clinical outcomes (greater accuracy, fewer and smaller scars, lower blood loss, less pain, reduced hospital stays, increased recovery times) compared to laparoscopic and open surgery. In highly specialist areas, where surgeons with the requisite skills are rare, robotic surgeons can also be employed remotely, allowing a surgeon to perform a procedure even when patient and surgeon are on opposite sides of the planet, potentially bringing world-class surgical care to underserved regions.

Robotic surgical systems have already transformed certain procedures by offering enhanced precision and visualisation, but the next wave of surgical robotics promises even greater benefits through increased autonomy and accessibility.

Robotic assistance

Beyond the operating room, assistive robots are beginning to support healthcare in other ways, helping patients with mobility limitations, delivering medications in hospitals, and even providing companionship to reduce isolation among elderly patients. While fully autonomous surgical robots remain largely theoretical, systems capable of handling specific surgical tasks under human supervision are advancing rapidly. These innovations could help address global shortages of surgical providers while standardising procedure quality across different settings. As costs decrease and capabilities increase, robotic assistance will likely become standard across a wider range of medical specialties, potentially democratising access to sophisticated surgical techniques that are currently available only at premier medical centres.

UV-C disinfection robots

Ultraviolet-C disinfection robots have begun to transform hospital infection control by automating the process of room sterilisation between patients. These autonomous machines emit powerful UV-C light that destroys the DNA of harmful microorganisms, including antibiotic-resistant bacteria and viruses that may survive traditional cleaning methods.

For hospital patients, this technology significantly reduces the risk of healthcare-associated infections that affect millions globally each year. The robots navigate patient rooms independently after conventional cleaning, reaching surfaces that might be missed during manual disinfection and eliminating pathogens without chemicals that can leave residues or trigger sensitivities. Most systems can disinfect a standard hospital room in ten to 15 minutes, improving turnover times without compromising safety. Around the globe, deployment has expanded beyond operating rooms to include patient rooms, emergency departments and other high-risk areas.

During the Covid-19 pandemic, many hospitals accelerated adoption of these systems to supplement manual cleaning protocols, with studies showing significant reductions in surface contamination (Pfleger et al 2025). Safety features prevent UV exposure to people, typically using motion sensors to shut down if someone enters during disinfection. While representing a significant investment, the technology has demonstrated cost-effectiveness through reduced infection rates and associated complications.

By consistently eliminating pathogens that conventional cleaning might miss, these robots address one of healthcare's most persistent challenges: preventing transmission of dangerous micro-organisms between vulnerable patients in shared environments.

Social robots for care of the elderly

The global ageing population presents unprecedented challenges for healthcare systems, with growing numbers of elderly people requiring assistance while facing social isolation. Social robots

– autonomous machines designed to interact with humans in emotionally intelligent ways – offer a potential solution, providing both practical support and companionship.

Already, relatively simple social robots are helping seniors remember to take medications, connecting them with family members through video calls and alerting caregivers to potential emergencies. More advanced models can engage in limited conversations, play cognitive games to maintain mental sharpness and even respond to emotional cues with appropriate expressions or statements. For families caring for elderly members, these robots can provide respite while ensuring loved ones are never truly alone. While the technology raises important ethical questions about the nature of care relationships, early research suggests many seniors form meaningful attachments to their robotic companions, viewing them as supportive presences rather than cold machines. As artificial intelligence and natural language processing improve, social robots will likely become more conversationally sophisticated and responsive to emotional nuances.

Though they won't replace human caregivers, these systems could become valuable members of elderly care teams, particularly in regions facing critical shortages of healthcare workers as demographic shifts continue to increase the proportion of older generations.

Immersive medical visualisation

This umbrella term captures a range of emerging technologies that create visual overlays and digital environments that enhance medical procedures and understanding through spatial computing and immersive visualisation environments, sometimes creating lifelike replicas of real situations.

Virtual and augmented reality

Imagine being able to practise complex surgery without any risk to the patient. Imagine being able to show patients what is wrong with them by taking them into their bodies to witness the problem first hand. Imagine conducting a consultation with a patient where information relating to that patient – personal data, diagnoses, treatment options – floats in the air in real time so it is no longer necessary to look it all up. This is the promise of virtual and augmented reality (VR/AR), which could potentially have a myriad of uses in healthcare.

VR allows clinicians to experience what life is actually like for patients, for example simulating the world of a wheelchair user or demonstrating how the world we perceive changes as we grow old. Today, VR is particularly starting to gain traction in mental healthcare, where patients can be exposed to what drives their anxieties and phobias in a safe, entirely virtual environment and learn how to deal with them.

Augmented reality (AR), where VR information is overlaid onto real life, is a growing trend that spans all industry sectors, but is particularly powerful in healthcare. AR applications are still in their infancy but initial use cases look set to be established in medical training. AR allows clinicians to see diagnoses and procedures in totally new ways, expanding both their knowledge and skills. AR also makes it possible to train more aspiring clinicians at once and in remote locations, helping alleviate the shortage of trained professionals around the world.

Surgical navigation systems

Surgical navigation systems function like GPS for surgeons, creating real-time digital maps of a patient's anatomy during procedures. These systems combine preoperative imaging with intraoperative tracking to show precisely where surgical instruments are located relative to critical structures like major blood vessels or nerves.

For patients undergoing complex surgeries, this technology reduces the risk of complications by helping surgeons avoid damaging these crucial areas of the anatomy, particularly in areas with limited visibility or abnormal anatomy due to tumours or previous surgeries. The systems are especially valuable in neurosurgery, where millimetre precision can mean the difference between successful treatment and devastating complications. Recent advances include augmented reality overlays that project imaging data directly onto surgeons' views of the patient through specialised headsets, eliminating the need to look away at screens during critical moments. AI integration enables these systems to identify anatomical structures automatically and alert surgeons to potential risks in real time.

In some areas, the technology has expanded from academic medical centres to community hospitals, making precision surgical approaches more widely available. While requiring significant investment and training, navigation systems reduce complications, decrease operating times and improve outcomes across multiple surgical specialties. By providing surgeons with enhanced visualisation and precision guidance, these systems represent one of the most significant advances in surgical technology of the past decade.

Digital twins for treatment planning

Digital twins (virtual replicas of physical objects or processes) are moving from industrial applications into healthcare, where they promise to revolutionise treatment planning and disease management. By creating detailed computational models of individual patients based on their unique anatomy, physiology and genetic make-up, doctors can simulate how different interventions might affect outcomes before attempting them in real life.

For complex surgeries, digital twins allow surgeons to practise procedures on virtual patients, identifying potential complications and optimising approaches before entering the operating room. The next generation of these systems will incorporate real-time data from wearable devices, continuously updating to reflect changes in patient condition and creating what amounts to a virtual medical dashboard for each individual – a powerful tool for both healthcare providers and patients themselves in making informed treatment decisions.

Digital twins for medication development

Digital twins technology has similarly revolutionised pharmaceutical research by creating virtual replicas of human physiological systems for medication testing. These sophisticated computer models simulate how drugs interact with specific organs or body systems, allowing researchers to predict efficacy and side effects before human trials begin.

The technology combines patient-specific data with advanced algorithms to create personalised biological models, enabling researchers to test thousands of potential drug compounds quickly and safely. Several major pharmaceutical companies have already integrated digital twins into their research pipelines, cutting years off traditional drug development timelines. For complex conditions such as heart disease, researchers can create virtual heart models reflecting different patient profiles to determine which medications might work best for specific genetic backgrounds or disease presentations. The technology has proven particularly valuable for rare diseases, where finding sufficient trial participants is challenging. By testing virtual patient populations, researchers can advance treatments that might otherwise never reach development due to market size limitations.

While still evolving, digital twins have already contributed to bringing several innovative treatments to market faster than would have been possible through conventional methods alone, representing one of the most significant shifts in how new medications are discovered and validated in decades (Ananth 2024).

Clinical support systems

As I have shown in this chapter so far, there are a vast number of emerging tools based on digital technologies entering the healthcare sphere. While some of these are being used to support and deliver complex medical procedures, other innovations are simply assisting with admin or are supporting clinicians to get to grips with a wide range of incoming data that might otherwise be hard to interpret. Day-to-day clinical practice isn't all cutting edge, but digital technologies can still play an important role.

Ambient clinical intelligence

The administrative burden of documentation represents one of the leading causes of clinician burnout, with doctors often spending more time on paperwork than with patients. Voice-assisted clinical documentation (or ambient) systems use natural language processing to transcribe conversations during appointments, automatically generating structured medical notes that integrate with electronic health records. Specialised microphones capture the clinical encounter, while sophisticated algorithms distinguish between speakers and identify medically relevant information for inclusion in the electronic health record.

For doctors, these systems promise to restore the focus on patient interaction rather than computer screens, potentially improving both job satisfaction and care quality. Patients benefit from more attentive providers who can maintain eye contact and observe subtle physical cues during consultations rather than typing. The technology also creates more comprehensive records by capturing details that might otherwise be forgotten in after-the-fact documentation. While current systems still require human review for accuracy, their capabilities are improving rapidly, with some able to identify key medical terms and suggest appropriate clinical codes.

Many health providers have implemented these systems, reporting improvements in physician satisfaction, consultation quality and documentation accuracy. Privacy protections include strict data encryption, patient consent procedures and the ability to pause recording for sensitive discussions.

As these tools mature, they'll likely expand beyond transcription to offer real-time clinical decision support (see following section), suggesting relevant tests or treatments based on the conversation content. By reducing administrative workload while improving documentation quality, voice assistance could help address the growing shortage of healthcare providers by allowing each clinician to care for more patients without sacrificing quality.

By addressing the documentation burden that consumes an estimated third of clinicians' time (Nuance 2022), ambient intelligence represents one of the most significant workflow innovations in modern clinical practice and, at the time of writing, is being rolled out in healthcare systems around the world at a significantly accelerated pace.

Augmented intelligence for clinical decision support

Rather than replacing human judgement, augmented intelligence systems aim to enhance it by providing clinicians with relevant information and evidence-based recommendations at the point of care. These systems integrate patient data from multiple sources with medical literature and clinical guidelines, helping doctors navigate increasingly complex treatment decisions.

For time-pressured clinicians, augmented intelligence can flag potential medication interactions, suggest appropriate diagnostic tests based on symptoms and identify patients who might benefit from preventative interventions. The technology is particularly valuable for primary care providers who must maintain knowledge across numerous specialties and keep pace with rapidly evolving medical evidence.

For patients, these systems reduce the risk of errors and ensure treatment decisions incorporate the latest research findings, regardless of where they receive care. Unlike automated systems that remove humans from the loop, augmented intelligence preserves physician autonomy while providing decision support, with the final judgement remaining in human hands.

As these tools become more sophisticated, they'll likely incorporate genetic information and social determinants of health alongside traditional medical data, offering truly comprehensive decision support.

By reducing cognitive burden on healthcare providers without replacing their critical thinking and empathy, augmented intelligence represents a balanced approach to healthcare technology that enhances human capabilities rather than attempting to supplant them.

Smart technologies

Patient care and comfort has seen a dramatic improvement across the healthcare spectrum due a new wave of smart technology products (ie devices that are designed to operate in a more intelligent, efficient and interconnected manner, typically integrating computing and telecommunication technology into objects that did not previously have such capabilities). Utilising connectivity and automation technologies, these tools can alleviate some of the pressure on the healthcare system while also putting power and control in the hands of patients. Industry-wide, there is now a trend toward smart technology implementation.

Smart technology products have been developed for hospital and home, and come in a variety of forms designed to increase efficiency and reduce risk.

In hospitals, smart beds now self-adjust to the correct pressure and support for each patient's circumstances. Smart monitors can observe a patient and take limited actions without a clinician being present.

In the home, as mentioned earlier in the chapter, smart devices can control insulin delivery for diabetes sufferers. Similarly, smart inhalers link via Bluetooth to smartphones and manage the delivery of asthma control medications, requiring less medicine overall and increasing the number of inhaler-free days.

Smart infusion pumps

Smart infusion pumps have transformed medication administration by adding digital safeguards to traditional intravenous delivery systems. These computerised devices contain comprehensive medication libraries with predetermined dosing limits and can integrate with electronic health records to verify orders against patient information.

For patients receiving intravenous medications, particularly high-risk drugs such as chemotherapy agents or blood thinners, these pumps dramatically reduce the risk of dangerous dosing errors. Should a nurse programme a dose outside safe parameters, the pump alerts them before administration begins. Most systems require documentation when limits are overridden, creating accountability and data for quality improvement. Advanced pumps can scan patient barcodes and medication barcodes, ensuring the right drug reaches the right patient.

Integration with electronic health records means the pumps automatically document medication administration, eliminating manual charting and potential transcription errors. Data collected from smart pumps helps hospitals identify recurring medication issues and improve safety protocols.

While implementation requires significant investment in both technology and staff training, the introduction of smart pumps as standard equipment in hospitals worldwide has driven a substantial reduction in serious medication errors. By adding multiple layers of digital verification to the medication administration process, these devices address one of the most persistent sources of preventable harm in healthcare: intravenous medication errors that affect hundreds of thousands of patients annually (Tariq et al 2024).

Smart hospitals and the internet of medical things

Building on the smart technology revolution, the hospital of the near future will be thoroughly connected, with sensors and devices communicating continuously to optimise patient care and operational efficiency. From smart beds to medication cabinets that track inventory in real time, the internet of medical things (IoMT) is transforming facility management and clinical workflows.

For patients, this connectivity translates to more attentive care without constant staff interruptions – vital signs trigger alerts when they fall outside normal ranges, while room conditions such as temperature and lighting adjust automatically to enhance healing and comfort. Smart hospitals are also implementing location tracking for equipment and personnel, reducing the time spent searching for necessary resources during emergencies.

Perhaps most significantly, these connected systems generate vast amounts of operational data that can identify inefficiencies and bottlenecks, helping administrators allocate resources more effectively. Interoperability, the ability for different digital healthcare systems to exchange information, is one of the main themes that will recur throughout this book. As interoperability standards evolve, it is likely that seamless information flow between devices from different manufacturers will become the norm, creating truly integrated care environments.

While the initial investment in smart hospital infrastructure is substantial, early adopters are already reporting improved patient outcomes and significant cost savings through optimised resource utilisation (Trustmarque 2025).

No longer science fiction…

While all the aforementioned digital technologies are in themselves ground-breaking, there are even more emerging technologies that could have potentially huge benefits for healthcare. Some of these would only have been dreamed of just a few years ago but are already advancing in leaps and bounds.

Brain–computer interfaces

Once confined to science fiction, brain–computer interfaces (BCIs) are increasingly becoming reality, offering hope for patients with neurological conditions that limit their ability to communicate or interact with their environment. These systems translate brain activity into digital commands, allowing direct control of computers, prosthetic limbs or other devices without physical movement.

For people with paralysis, BCIs offer the possibility of regained independence through mind-controlled wheelchairs or robotic assistants. Current clinical applications focus primarily on communication, allowing completely paralysed individuals to type messages, browse the internet or control environmental features such as lights and television. Similarly, patients with locked-in syndrome, who are fully conscious but unable to move or communicate, may regain their voices through BCI systems that translate thought patterns into speech.

While invasive BCIs requiring surgical implantation are currently limited to research settings, non-invasive alternatives using external sensors are advancing rapidly, though with lower signal resolution. The technology faces significant technical and ethical challenges, including questions about data security and cognitive privacy. However, preliminary results from clinical trials have been promising enough to attract substantial investment from both medical research institutions and technology companies (eg Johns Hopkins Medicine 2024).

BCI technology represents one of the most direct connections between human cognition and digital systems, offering hope for patients previously unable to interact with their environment and raising fascinating questions about the future relationship between minds and machines as capabilities continue to expand.

Within the next decade, BCIs are likely to become standard treatments for certain neurological conditions, while more sophisticated applications – including memory enhancement and direct brain-to-brain communication – remain active areas of research that could eventually transform how humans interact with technology and each other.

Nanotechnology for targeted drug delivery

Conventional medication delivery often treats the entire body to address problems in specific locations, leading to unnecessary side effects and limiting effective dosages. Nanotechnology offers a solution through microscopically small carriers that can transport drugs directly to diseased cells while sparing healthy tissue.

In cancer treatment, nanoparticles can be designed to recognise and bind to tumour cells, delivering chemotherapy agents precisely where needed and dramatically reducing damage to healthy tissues. This targeted approach allows for higher effective doses at the disease site while minimising systemic exposure. Beyond cancer, nano delivery systems are being developed for conditions ranging from macular degeneration (gradual loss of central vision) to atherosclerosis (a build-up of arterial plaque), where medications need to reach specific tissues that are difficult to target with conventional approaches. Some advanced nanoparticles can even respond to environmental triggers, releasing their payloads only under certain conditions like specific pH levels or enzyme presence.

While regulatory approval processes for nanomedicines remain rigorous, several products have already reached clinical use, with many more in development pipelines. As manufacturing techniques improve and costs decrease, nanomedicine will likely become standard for conditions where precise drug delivery dramatically improves the benefit–risk profile, potentially transforming treatment for diseases that currently require accepting significant side effects as the price of effective therapy.

Quantum computing in drug discovery

The process of developing new medications traditionally takes years and billions of dollars, with many promising compounds failing in late-stage trials. Quantum computing, which leverages quantum mechanical phenomena to perform calculations impossible for conventional computers, could dramatically accelerate this process by simulating molecular interactions with unprecedented accuracy.

For patients with conditions that lack effective treatments, quantum-enabled drug discovery could bring new therapies to market years faster than conventional approaches. The technology is particularly promising for complex diseases involving protein misfolding, such as Alzheimer's and Parkinson's, where conventional computing struggles to model the relevant biochemical processes. Quantum computing could also revolutionise precision medicine by efficiently analysing how genetic variations affect drug responses, potentially predicting which medications will work best for individual patients. While functional quantum computers with sufficient power for comprehensive drug simulations are still developing, hybrid approaches combining quantum and classical computing are already showing promise in preliminary research (eg Swayne 2025). Major pharmaceutical companies are investing heavily in the technology, recognising its potential to transform research and development (R&D) productivity.

As quantum computing matures over the next decade, it could fundamentally change how new treatments are developed, potentially addressing diseases that have resisted conventional research approaches for decades.

4 The impact of AI

Full disclosure: the last chapter was developed with the significant support of artificial intelligence large language models (LLMs). I used AI to help me research all of the latest technologies used in healthcare today and provide information and sources on each. For years, I have been subscribing to email newsletters on digital healthcare to provide me with material in preparation for this book. Suddenly, rather than laboriously trudging through them all, I was able to use AI to analyse their content en masse and provide me with summaries and lists of recurring topics. I compiled all the technologies I found on a whiteboard – semi-randomly – and then uploaded a photograph of the whiteboard to an AI tool and asked it to group them into themes. It was (largely) able to read my scrawly handwriting (although 'leaf patient fracking' was clearly a valiant but failed attempt) and the result was commendable. However, the LLM did also advise me – quite correctly – that there were a number of ways that the technologies could be grouped thematically and that many of them fitted into multiple categories. I was also warned that digital healthcare was evolving rapidly with new innovations and applications constantly emerging. Basically, I needed to get this book written or it would quickly become out of date!

Today, AI is everywhere and we have only just begun to exploit its potential. The healthcare sector was very guarded when the internet arrived and it has been equally reluctant to dive headlong into broad AI adoption, concerned that any advice delivered out of an opaque black box essentially carries too much risk for both clinicians and patients. Disappointingly, healthcare leaders seem to believe that clinicians will simply do what AI says without thinking for themselves or challenging AI output based on their own training, knowledge and experience. Personally, at this point in the AI revolution, I would prefer to see clinicians working in collaboration with AI, challenging each other and both learning from the experience. But at the time of writing, that is considered too risky.

Not surprisingly, AI is gradually finding its way into many of the technologies I have already discussed, but for now I will provide just a few additional examples.

Medical imaging analysis

AI algorithms excel at analysing medical images, from X-rays, MRIs and CT scans to ultrasounds. Deep learning models can detect subtle abnormalities that might be missed by human eyes, helping radiologists identify potential cancers, fractures, haemorrhages and other conditions with greater accuracy and speed. These systems are particularly valuable for early detection of diseases such as breast cancer, lung nodules and stroke, where prompt intervention can significantly improve outcomes.

Artificial intelligence for diagnosis

AI diagnostic tools are expanding beyond radiology into pathology, dermatology and other specialties. For patients, this means more accurate diagnoses without waiting for specialist appointments, which is particularly valuable in regions with doctor shortages. The technology doesn't aim to replace doctors but rather to serve as a powerful assistant, flagging concerning images for human review and reducing the risk of missed diagnoses. Recent studies suggest that AI systems can already match or exceed human experts in detecting certain conditions (Milmo 2025), though the final medical decisions will remain in human hands for the foreseeable future.

Diagnosing retinal disease

As a specific example, artificial intelligence systems for diagnosing retinal diseases have moved from research to routine clinical use, analysing images from eye examinations to detect conditions such as diabetic retinopathy and macular degeneration, with accuracy matching or exceeding human specialists. These systems use deep-learning algorithms trained on millions of retinal images to identify subtle changes invisible to the unaided eye.

For diabetic patients who require regular eye screening to prevent blindness, AI-based systems have proven particularly valuable, especially in regions with shortages of ophthalmologists. Several approved systems can now grade the severity of diabetic retinopathy and recommend appropriate follow-up timing based on standard clinical guidelines. The technology has expanded eye-screening capabilities to primary-care settings and even mobile clinics, bringing specialist-level diagnostics to communities without ready access to eye care professionals. Recent advances include systems that can predict cardiovascular risk from retinal images, recognising patterns associated with heart disease that human clinicians might not connect to eye findings. While AI can't replace comprehensive eye examinations, it has become an efficient first-line screening tool, allowing specialists to focus their attention on patients with confirmed abnormalities. The technology represents one of the most successful clinical implementations of artificial intelligence to date, demonstrating how AI can expand access to specialist-level diagnostics while improving efficiency in mainstream medical practice.

AI-powered virtual health assistants

These AI-driven tools support patients through digital communication, offering personalised health information, medication reminders and appointment scheduling. They can also answer patients' questions and provide tailored health tips, improving patient engagement and adherence to treatment plans. These virtual assistants can be integrated into mobile apps and other digital platforms, making healthcare more accessible. For example, a virtual assistant could remind a patient to take their medication and provide information about potential side effects.

In the next few years, there will no doubt be another book to write just on the use of AI in healthcare settings. Advances are being made all the time, potential risks are being identified at an equally exponential rate and it is almost impossible to predict where we will end up in the short term. Long term, however, and assuming there isn't the AI apocalypse feared by many, I am sure AI will become an omniscient and ubiquitous presence in healthcare that we will simply take for granted, permeating everything and making data-driven healthcare second nature. In the short term, however, what AI can offer will only be as good as the data available to it. And as we will see, there is still much work to do on preparing the foundations before AI can be safely and productively unleashed to solve our healthcare problems.

5 The rise of data in healthcare

Having examined the key technological and engineering advances driving healthcare in the preceding chapters, I will now review those developments that are purely or primarily related to data technologies. Separating the new healthcare technological landscape into data and non-data categories is a somewhat arbitrary process as a superficial review of the technologies just summarised will immediately reveal a huge dependence on data at their foundations. Ultimately, everything digital can be reduced down to 1s and 0s.

For example, personalised medicine and genetic science essentially deal with vast libraries of data that will be created and used to develop treatments. Similarly, telehealth at its core represents the transmission of data; 3D printing relies on patterns constructed of data; smart devices, wearables and biosensors capture data; and virtual worlds are made solely out of data. What distinguishes the aforementioned technologies, however, is that they are more than data; there's a lot more science and engineering going on.

In the journey toward data-driven healthcare and the next generation of the patient care record, the data I refer to from now on includes all the information that is captured and stored as the patient navigates the healthcare system. This can include simple demographic information such as age and gender, but also complex data such as vital signs and genomic information. The important thing to note here is that this data too is being captured in a shifting environment of general data technologies that are becoming increasingly powerful, clever and ubiquitous.

Big data

Big data refers to extremely large and complex datasets that cannot be effectively managed, processed or analysed using traditional data-processing methods or tools. It is characterised by what are commonly known as the 'Three Vs':

- **Volume:** The sheer quantity of data, often measured in terabytes, petabytes or even exabytes. (An exabyte is a billion gigabytes.)
- **Velocity:** The speed at which new data is generated and needs to be processed, often in real time or near real time.
- **Variety:** The diverse types and formats of data, including structured data (such as databases), semi-structured data (such as XML or JSON files) and unstructured data (such as text documents, images, videos and social media posts). It is also possible for unstructured data to contain structured data (eg the use of a code within free text).

Some industry definitions add additional Vs, such as Veracity (the reliability and accuracy of data) and Value (the ability to turn data into useful insights).

Big data, and the ability to work with it, lies behind the success of social media platforms such as Facebook and X (formerly Twitter) and ecommerce sites such as Amazon. In healthcare specifically, big data theoretically encompasses everything from electronic health records and medical imaging to genomic sequences, insurance claims, patient-generated health data from wearables and social determinants of health. However, while there has been an explosion of healthcare data over the past decade, coupled with corresponding advances in computing power and machine-learning algorithms, to date these various components have rarely been brought together to truly create big healthcare datasets. The challenge and opportunity lie in integrating these diverse data sources to generate meaningful insights that can improve patient outcomes, reduce costs and enhance the overall healthcare experience.

At a more local level, big data techniques have been used in a number of practical, high-impact applications. Predictive analytics now help to identify patients at risk for hospital readmissions or disease complications before symptoms appear. Precision medicine initiatives use genetic and molecular data to tailor treatments to individual patients, moving beyond one-size-fits-all approaches. Population health management benefits from comprehensive data analysis to identify vulnerable communities and target interventions effectively. Meanwhile, operational efficiency has improved through capacity planning, resource allocation and supply chain optimisation informed by data science. Perhaps most visibly during the Covid-19 pandemic, big data enabled rapid disease surveillance, contact tracing and vaccine development, demonstrating both the potential and necessity of a robust healthcare data infrastructure in addressing public health challenges.

Digital phenotypes

One area of great potential for data-driven healthcare is the construction of individualised digital phenotypes for patients. If personalised medicine is set to customise treatments across a range of physical conditions, then digital phenotyping could be considered an extended approach that would be particularly useful in mental health.

While precision medicine uses a patient's *genotype* to direct interventions, the same patient's *phenotype* represents the expression of those genes in the environment. Examples include observable characteristics such as height, weight, hair and eye colour. The range of possibilities is determined by an individual's genotype but the actual expression of those genes (brown eyes, fair hair) results from a combination of their genetic make-up and their surroundings. Genotypes are directly inherited from parents but phenotypes are not, since the environment introduces variables not associated with ancestry. As a result, while genotypes are fixed for life, phenotypes can differ, even between identical twins (if, for example, they adopt different diets), and can also change over time.

A *digital* phenotype extends this idea beyond gene-driven characteristics to details about a person that can be measured and recorded as data, which these days is pretty much anything. So, while a digital phenotype includes an individual's genome and corresponding genetically driven phenotype, it can also incorporate a digital representation of their behaviours, health or social status and traits. Some definitions limit the digital phenotype to data that can be collected on digital devices, but I believe this is short sighted. For example, wealth has long been shown to correlate with nutritional health. Similarly, while it might be possible to design devices that count how many cigarettes or units of alcohol someone consumes, it would generally be considered to be overengineering against the alternative of simply counting, yet both of these substances are massively influential in determining health status.

It is true, however, that many different types of *relevant* health-related data can be recorded as they are observed through interactions with technology. Collecting a wide variety of data associated with a patient enables clinicians to build a digital profile that has the potential to be used to direct treatment decisions. The variety of data sources is expanding and today includes smartphones and wearables, not just to gather the data entered or captured by patients deliberately, but also to track device usage and movements. GPS and accelerometer data, for example, have proven useful in measuring levels of physical activity and abnormal or involuntary movements. Analysing selfies or tone of voice from small snippets of conversation can pick up a patient's mood. Tracking numbers of phone calls and text messages, including the lengths of those messages, may also prove invaluable in flagging a patient's deteriorating emotional state. With the patient's permission, all of these could be captured without compromising a patient's confidentiality or exposing the content of any call or messages.

Unlike traditional phenotypes that describe observable physical or biochemical characteristics, these components of digital phenotypes represent patterns in data that might reveal underlying health states or behaviours. And this is why digital phenotypes are particularly useful in mental health. For example, changes in communication frequency, sleep patterns, mobility or typing dynamics might all indicate shifts in psychological wellbeing.

These digital markers could be collected passively and continuously, providing richer longitudinal data than that typically available through occasional clinical assessments. At a population level, this data provides researchers and clinicians with the potential to use digital phenotypes to better understand, predict and potentially intervene in various health conditions, particularly in mental or neurodegenerative disorders and chronic disease management.

As I will show, the digital phenotype is an essential component of data-driven healthcare but there is a compromise to be made. The more variables that are introduced into the phenotype, the more personalised the treatment recommendations. However, it can quickly become so personalised that treatment recommendations are essentially being derived from a sample of one, and are therefore not data-driven recommendations at all. This is why I highlighted the word *relevant* at the beginning of the last but one paragraph. Depending on the context of the healthcare intervention in question, if it is not relevant to include whether a person has blue, green or brown eyes, then that observation should be excluded from the analysis of the phenotype. That said, we are fast entering a world where the analytic algorithms are more than capable of determining which factors are relevant or not, and therefore which can be ignored, even from massive datasets. Consequently, it is inevitable that the range of data included in digital phenotypes will only increase over time, possibly exponentially.

Predictive analytics and early intervention

The vast amounts of health data generated through electronic records, wearable devices and genetic testing create opportunities for predictive analytics to identify patients at risk before they develop serious symptoms. Using machine-learning algorithms, healthcare systems can now analyse patterns across thousands of variables to flag individuals who might benefit from preventative interventions.

Some hospitals are already using these systems to predict which patients are at high risk for readmission or complications, allowing care teams to allocate resources more effectively. The potential applications extend far beyond hospital walls – community health programmes could identify neighbourhood-level risk factors, while primary care practices could proactively reach out to patients showing early warning signs of chronic disease. As these systems become more sophisticated, they'll likely incorporate social determinants of health such as housing stability and food access, recognising that medical outcomes are influenced by factors outside traditional healthcare settings. The ethical implementation of predictive analytics requires careful attention to potential biases in the underlying data, ensuring that technological advances don't exacerbate existing healthcare disparities. When properly deployed, however, these tools promise to shift healthcare focus from treating established disease to preventing it, potentially saving both lives and healthcare costs.

Population healthcare

Integrating patient records across diverse healthcare settings would create a comprehensive view of individual health journeys, enabling providers to identify patterns, gaps in care and opportunities for intervention that might be missed when data remains siloed. When clinicians are able to access complete medical histories – including primary care visits, specialist consultations, emergency department encounters, hospitalisations and pharmacy records – they can then make more informed decisions, avoid redundant testing, prevent adverse medication interactions and coordinate care more effectively. This holistic approach is particularly beneficial for managing chronic conditions and complex cases requiring multiple providers.

At a population level, this consolidated data – anonymised and aggregated – becomes an invaluable resource for public health initiatives, allowing analysts to gain valuable insights into the effectiveness of different treatments and to identify health trends, disparities in care access and social determinants affecting health outcomes. Healthcare organisations would then have the information to enable them to implement targeted preventive measures, allocate resources more efficiently to areas of greatest need, introduce new policies and develop evidence-based protocols that address population-specific health challenges, all contributing to continual improvement in population health and wellbeing. Additionally, researchers can leverage this comprehensive data to evaluate treatment effectiveness across diverse patient groups, accelerating medical advances and contributing to more equitable, cost-effective healthcare delivery systems that improve outcomes for entire communities.

6 The care record

All the technologies described in Chapters 3 and 4 have one thing in common: they produce data, sometimes lots of it. But they collect it in different places, at different times, and if it was simply left where it was produced then a complete picture of a patient's healthcare history would be scattered over a myriad of different systems.

From a data perspective, the healthcare record *ideally* stands as the foundational cornerstone of patient care, serving as the primary repository where an individual's complete medical journey is meticulously documented. From the initial symptoms that prompt a visit to the latest diagnostic test results, treatment plans, medication histories and ongoing progress notes, every piece of health-related information finds its home within this vital repository. Far more than a mere collection of facts, the healthcare record provides a longitudinal narrative, ensuring that comprehensive and up-to-date data is readily accessible to clinicians, enabling informed decision making and continuity of care throughout a patient's life.

That's the ideal. The reality today is quite different.

A brief history

When it comes to understanding the landscape of present day healthcare data and records management, I believe it is necessary to first rehearse where it started. While the evolution of systems around the world will be quite similar, I will primarily refer to that experienced in the UK National Health Service (NHS) as a typical example.

In the 1980s, patient administration systems (PASs) were introduced in hospitals across the NHS, due to emerging requirements to routinely collect administrative data and a recognition that electronic records were a better long-term solution than pen and paper. The PAS was fundamentally about scheduling and tracking and contained little to no clinical information. It was an administrative system for patient demographic information, patient master index (PMI), admitting, transferring and discharging patients (ADT), information on inpatient/outpatient (eg referrals/bookings) and activity to manage things such as waiting times, bed management or order communications (OCS) for requesting diagnostics and drugs etc. Then, in the mid-late nineties, electronic patient record (EPR) and departmental systems began to be implemented, which dealt with the clinical information specifically required to replace paper medical records and facilitate good care. The PAS and EPR systems were naturally integrated – the PAS usually updating the EPR. Over time, as both PASs and EPRs have developed, the line between traditional PAS systems and modern EPRs is less clear. Whether addressed by one or two systems, however, the needs of healthcare providers are still the same today: timely and accurate information – both administrative and clinical – must be routinely captured and accessible in order to coordinate safe and high-quality care.

In the NHS, secondary care (acute hospitals) are now well catered for in regard to EPRs. There are many suppliers providing technology for this sector, although as we entered the current decade, Matthew Gould, the then CEO of NHSX, a department of NHS England tasked with driving digital transformation, claimed 10 per cent of trusts remained 'largely paper-based' with 'a whole lot more that are only semi-digitised' (Carding 2021). The requirement for accurate and timely information is, however, not restricted to hospitals.

In the UK, primary care has, over time, developed a duopoly of patient record systems – Optum (formerly EMIS) and SystmOne. This is repeatedly challenged by the government, which is looking for better products and choice; though, like most advancements in health tech, I don't think this will be a quick fix and there remain significant barriers for new entrants to the market.

Community and mental health services have been traditionally underserved both in regard to budget and in the drive to implement EPRs and other supporting IT infrastructure.

For years, the debate around patient record system strategy has oscillated between a best of breed (niche, differentiated) departmental system approach and a monolithic, whole-organisation, one-size-fits-all generic EPR solution. Both have their strengths and weaknesses, which I will explore further in Chapter 8 (Theme 5). In the early 2000s, a mix of both models began to emerge across the country.

In 2005, an organisation called Connecting for Health was created to deliver the NHS National Programme for IT (NPfIT). This initiative recognised the need for IT systems and infrastructure to support the health service, and the large variation in systems and success across the country. This ambitious programme achieved many noteworthy things, such as delivery of the national Spine (providing backbone systems for other systems to connect to), N3 Network (a private internet for the NHS), NHSmail, Choose and Book, Secondary Uses Service and Picture Archiving and Communications Service. One key objective of NPfIT, however, was to deliver a single EPR system across England – from a small number of suppliers split into territories. When it was finally dismantled in 2011, NPfIT cost £10 billion. Only a handful of EPR systems were implemented – and with far less functionality than expected. You can find a summary on the failures of the programme on the National Audit Office website together with a useful breakdown of project costs and realised benefits (NAO 2011).

There are multiple reasons why this is an important context for this book: the one-size-fits-all approach has proven problematic, things move slowly in health tech, and the NPfIT programme and its many failures continue to influence the way people now think about technology in healthcare.

Providing one system that fulfils the purpose of all clinical specialties is difficult. Even with multi-million-pound contracts and almost a decade of negotiations and development, this was not successfully achieved. More success has been had outside the national programme, but this one-size-fits-all approach has not provided the best clinical solution for any speciality – it simply provides an acceptable minimum standard to everyone. Contracts that were signed as part of NPfIT have only recently started coming up for re-tender as they typically run for ten years with options to extend. Many of these systems are still in place, even if there is dissatisfaction with their performance, as moving suppliers is complex and costly. Once embedded in an NHS organisation, technology is difficult to displace, and for that reason the NHS deals with a huge issue of legacy systems that hamper progress as a whole. NPfIT was an attempt at a common, national approach, and for those who worked in the NHS at the time, the impact of this programme will not quickly be forgotten. The failure of the national programme to deliver what it promised – despite the significant investment – did a huge amount of damage to how clinicians and informatics professionals working in the health sector feel about health tech and the relationship between the NHS and suppliers.

In recent years, the emergence of new technology and shared interoperability standards means that health services should no longer have to sacrifice a specialist system in order to have all their records in one place. The generic one-size-fits-all EPR systems that do everything but nothing very well should no longer be the only option for specialist clinical services wanting to excel at the service they deliver.

However, despite the difficulties of the monolithic system approach, there remains a mentality among some of those procuring NHS IT that they want everything on one system as it makes their lives easier, and 'no one got fired for buying [Rio/Cerner/Epic]'. But trust-wide deployments of generic EPR systems are hugely costly and disruptive, not least for different departments trying to map its features onto their workflows. No NHS trust chief information officer wants to do more than one of those in their tenure. This is both a threat and an opportunity; very occasional wholesale deployments reduce the risks associated with multiple system changes while small, incremental deployments of more flexible and interoperable solutions will avoid the need for whole organisation migrations from big EPR to big EPR, while offering more tailored solutions to each clinical team and integrated records available in a virtual 'all in one place'.

How this ecosystem evolves is still being debated. It will inevitably emerge over time through a combination of innovation and collaboration between the NHS, suppliers and universal interoperability standards.

The procurement landscape is also changing. It may be that healthcare IT is increasingly procured at a regional level rather than trust level and via major procurement frameworks. Both could drive constraints on purchasing decisions and system procurements could become fewer but larger as a result.

At the same time, healthcare is looking to embrace all that new disciplines in data science have to offer in order to drive efficient, personalised, tailored care, resulting in improved health outcomes. This will require a sea change in the type, completeness, quality and structure of data that is collected in health record systems.

A universally hated industry

While over the past decade or so patient record systems have emerged that have been lauded by their users, the norm is currently for the majority of legacy systems used globally in healthcare today to be found wanting. Healthcare IT is often criticised by users and customers for several key reasons:

- ❖ **Poor usability**: Many healthcare IT systems, particularly electronic health record (EHR) systems, have interfaces that do not replicate clinical workflows. Physicians frequently complain about excessive clicking, unintuitive navigation and interfaces that interrupt rather than enhance patient care.
- ❖ **Fragmentation:** Healthcare systems rarely communicate well with each other. The lack of interoperability between different providers' systems means that patient data doesn't

flow smoothly, creating information silos that frustrate both clinicians and patients.
- **Implementation challenges:** Healthcare organisations often struggle with expensive, time-consuming implementations that disrupt operations and require extensive staff retraining.
- **Prioritisation of administrative needs:** Many systems were built primarily to optimise billing and regulatory compliance rather than clinical care, creating a fundamental misalignment with how healthcare professionals actually work.
- **Change resistance meets poor change management:** Healthcare practitioners are inherently conservative about adopting new technologies (for good reason – lives are at stake), but this is compounded by IT vendors who often provide inadequate training and support.
- **High costs with unclear return on investment (ROI):** Healthcare IT systems typically require substantial financial investment, but the benefits in terms of improved care quality or efficiency aren't always apparent to front-line users.

This widespread dissatisfaction has created something of a vicious cycle where frustration with current systems makes adopting newer, potentially better solutions even more challenging. The problem is exacerbated because legacy systems – built on what would now be considered ancient technology – do have the advantage of having the most bells and whistles. Functionality in newer systems can be quite limited, even if the technology it is built on has more potential to expand into the future. This trade-off can be quite perplexing for customers, with the result that doing nothing often seems the best option. Getting it wrong can be an expensive mistake and healthcare systems are generally not funded at a level where investments in uncertainty can be entertained.

Patients too can get drawn into the debate and find the systems inadequate to meet their needs. Access to basic functions such as appointment booking – now an everyday expectation on, say, a hotel booking site – are mostly found wanting in healthcare. Transparency of patient records or even allowing patients to add their own thoughts to them is a rarity. Similarly, outcome measurement as reported by patients desperate to feed back their experience into the system can be almost impossible to achieve, even when arguably this should be the most important piece of information sought by clinicians.

None of these problems are due to technical challenges. Developments in digital technology have overcome most of the hurdles. The challenges that remain are largely commercial, political, ethical and legal. These are clearly not insubstantial.

Patient safety

Patient safety must be the cornerstone of all digital patient record systems. While efficiency, cost savings and data analytics offer compelling benefits, these considerations should never supersede minimising the risks to patients. When healthcare systems prioritise patient safety, they create a foundation where critical information is accessible, accurate and actionable at the point of care. This enables clinicians to make informed decisions that directly impact patient outcomes, avoiding medication errors, missed diagnoses and treatment delays that can lead to preventable harm.

The consequences of deprioritising safety in healthcare system design can be devastating. Systems that value convenience or administrative efficiency over safety features may introduce new types of errors through poor interface design, alert fatigue or inadequate data validation. Research has consistently shown that poorly implemented systems can contribute to patient harm through information fragmentation, workflow disruptions and cognitive overload for healthcare providers. Every design decision in these systems should begin with the question, 'How does this protect patients from harm?'

Ultimately, patient safety as the primary concern aligns all other objectives in healthcare information systems. When safety drives system development, it naturally improves clinical workflow efficiency, enhances data quality and builds trust among both providers and patients. Regulatory frameworks increasingly recognise this hierarchy of priorities, but technology developers, healthcare organisations and policymakers must continually reaffirm that no feature, financial consideration or convenience factor should compromise the fundamental obligation to first do no harm.

Data standards

Data and communication standards are the bedrock of a truly joined-up healthcare service. They enable seamless information flow between disparate systems and providers, breaking down silos. This ensures clinicians have a holistic view of patient history, leading to more informed decisions and safer care. Standardisation streamlines workflows, reduces errors from manual data entry and facilitates efficient care coordination across different settings. Ultimately, these standards empower a more integrated, responsive and patient-centric healthcare experience.

Though it has been a painful process, with many regimes for common data standards rising and falling, some have made it to international status and been adopted by many countries. Though not an exhaustive list, these include:

- ❖ **HL7 (Health Level Seven):** A set of international standards for the transfer of clinical and administrative data between software applications used by various healthcare providers. However, different versions and implementation variations limit seamless interoperability.
- ❖ **FHIR (Fast Healthcare Interoperability Resources):** A newer, more modern standard from HL7 designed to improve interoperability through the use of application programming interfaces (APIs, which enable different software systems to interact with each other) and web-based technologies. Adoption is growing but not yet universal.
- ❖ **SNOMED CT (Systematised Nomenclature of Medicine – Clinical Terms):** A comprehensive clinical vocabulary used for coding clinical findings, diagnoses, procedures, etc. Widespread and consistent use of SNOMED CT can significantly improve data consistency.
- ❖ **ICD-10 (International Classification of Diseases, 10th Revision):** A standard for coding diagnoses and procedures,

primarily used for billing and statistical purposes. While widely adopted for these purposes, its granularity may not always be sufficient for detailed clinical data exchange.
- ❖ **DICOM (Digital Imaging and Communications in Medicine):** A standard for handling, storing, printing and transmitting medical images. Relatively well adopted within radiology but may not be consistently integrated with other systems.

Any attempt at true data-driven healthcare will be critically dependent on organisations agreeing and adopting common standards for coding and data exchange. And as you will see, standardised data recording will in turn be absolutely key to unleashing the power locked within care pathways to improve both efficiency and outcomes.

Patient-held records

The fragmented nature of healthcare information remains a significant barrier to coordinated care, with patient records often scattered across multiple providers and systems. To overcome this challenge, in the emerging future of healthcare data management, patients may become the primary custodians of their own medical information through personal health record (PHR) systems. These secure digital vaults could allow individuals to store their complete medical histories, from lab results and imaging studies to medication lists and clinical notes, on encrypted personal devices or cloud platforms accessible via biometric authentication. Such patient-centred approaches would empower individuals to grant temporary, granular access to healthcare providers across different facilities as needed, eliminating fragmentation of records between disparate systems.

This paradigm shift would fundamentally alter the healthcare data landscape, transforming patients from passive recipients of care to active partners in managing their health information. Wearable devices and home health-monitoring tools could automatically supplement these records with real-time health data, creating comprehensive health profiles that move seamlessly with patients throughout their lives and across healthcare systems, regardless of insurance changes or relocation to new communities.

In the future, we might see patients carrying their complete medical histories on smartphone apps, granting temporary access to healthcare providers as needed. This shift would not only improve care coordination but could also empower patients to take a more active role in managing their health by providing a comprehensive view of their medical information.

Blockchain for secure health records

Blockchain technology – a secure, decentralised digital ledger system – offers a potential solution to any privacy or security concerns associated with patient-held records by creating an immutable record of medical information that patients can control and share as needed.

By giving patients ownership of their health data while maintaining rigorous security, blockchain could eliminate delays in transferring records between facilities, reduce medical errors caused by incomplete information and prevent unauthorised access to sensitive details. The technology could prove particularly valuable during emergencies, when quick access to accurate information about allergies, medications and medical history can be life saving.

Although blockchain technology arrived with the advent of Bitcoin, it has been very slow to find a foothold in healthcare despite these apparently obvious advantages. Several pilot projects are exploring blockchain applications in healthcare, though challenges around system interoperability and regulatory compliance must be addressed before widespread adoption.

Digital health passports and immunity credentials

The global Covid-19 pandemic accelerated development of digital health credentials that securely store and verify vaccination status, test results and other health information. While initially focused on Covid, these systems are evolving into comprehensive health passports that could transform how medical information is shared across borders and between healthcare systems.

For travellers and patients seeking care outside their home regions, digital health passports offer a secure way to demonstrate vaccination status, medication histories or chronic conditions without carrying paper records that can be lost or damaged. The technology might finally find a use for blockchain or use other secure verification systems to ensure information cannot be falsified while giving individuals control over who can access their data and for what purpose. Beyond travel, these systems could streamline access to healthcare services by securely sharing relevant information with providers, eliminating redundant paperwork and reducing administrative burden. The implementation challenges are significant, requiring international standards and careful attention to privacy concerns, particularly for sensitive health information. However, the pandemic demonstrated both the feasibility and value of such systems when properly designed. As development continues, it is likely that the use of health passports will expand to include broader medical information while maintaining strong privacy protections, potentially creating truly portable health records that follow individuals throughout their lives regardless of where they receive care.

7 Data-driven healthcare

If you woke up one morning feeling unwell, in pain or struggling mentally, wouldn't it be wonderful if you could enter a pile of data into a computer and instantly receive a list of options for treatment together with predictions for the likely outcomes you'll achieve with each? You'd select one (which may be to go and see a professional clinician or therapist) and embark on a journey back to full health with an expectation of how well that should go and how long it will take. This is possible because you are not the first person to have done this. Many hundreds and thousands of people before you have had similar mornings and followed exactly the same process. In fact, it is because of them that you are able to do this too, and why the predictions for different treatments will be highly accurate – and likely even more accurate for you than it was for them. This, in essence, is the vision for data-driven healthcare.

But let's rewind a little. Imagine for a moment that this very morning you presented yourself to the healthcare profession with that new ailment. Maybe you overdid things in the garden and strained your lower back. Maybe you've started developing weekly migraines for no discernible reason. Perhaps your knees have begun to feel unstable as you try to keep pace with your son or daughter on the squash court. Or maybe you've become overwhelmed with anxiety and depression from the stresses that life has thrown at you.

Whatever has brought you to this place, the salient point is that you've recognised that you need help and desire to be taken on a journey back to full health, or as much of it as you can achieve. This is then what would have typically happened. The clinician would first of all have checked your registration details, or if this is a first referral, have registered you on their system, which means taking down an array of demographic details such as gender, age, ethnicity, where you live, your profession and aspects of your previous medical history. This is the information about you that doesn't really change and is therefore not necessary to collect if you are presenting for a second time, albeit for different reasons than the time before.

Having established who you are, the clinician then needs to establish and record why you think you're here. This is initiated by a 'referral', which in turn initiates an 'episode' of care. The information collected now relates only to your current circumstances, such as your presenting problem, where you've come from (eg if you've been referred by your GP or signposted by another healthcare service) and current life situation (eg pregnant, employed, smoker, height, weight etc). Referral information can and often does change from episode to episode, especially if those episodes are about completely different things.

Next, the clinician will supplement this information with some form of assessment, which may involve more questions and form filling, but may equally include diagnostic tests such as X-rays, ECGs, bloods, etc. This information taken together (registration, referral and assessment) comprises your profile for your current episode of care and, if the data is collected systematically and in a standardised form, makes up the basic digital phenotype referred to in Chapter 5.

All of the above is what every patient experiences in almost every healthcare setting in almost every country the world over. What a clinician typically does next is use all of that information to determine the best course of treatment (aka patient journey) based on their individual knowledge and experience. And why wouldn't they do that? After all, that's what they've been trained for and that's why we went to see them in the first place. But here's the interesting bit. What they won't ever do is go and find all the other patients like you (ie who have a similar digital phenotype/profile), review what treatment pathways they followed and what outcomes were achieved, and use *that* data to suggest the best treatment pathway for you.

In some ways, this is no different to what the legal profession does when they search through historical case law to inform predictions about how the current case will go. Precedents matter. But in healthcare, the big difference is that we are not just trying to find that one case that went our way but instead seek out the largest volume of interventions that have resulted in positive outcomes for previous patients (though for a very rare presentation, it might be that just finding that one similar historical case among millions will be the discovery that makes the difference). Data-driven healthcare, then, is primarily about using historical data on a massive scale to improve outcomes.

Healthcare interventions, quite rightly, are evidence based – or should be. Most treatments have been subjected to prolonged double-blind, randomised clinical trials before they are ever let loose on the wider public. Data-driven healthcare does not replace the need for these, but once a treatment has been judged effective and safe in general, data-driven techniques can be used to provide more clarity around which of the safe treatments available are most effective for different patient cohorts.

Here again is the diagram I shared in the first chapter: the simple equation that defines what data-driven healthcare is all about.

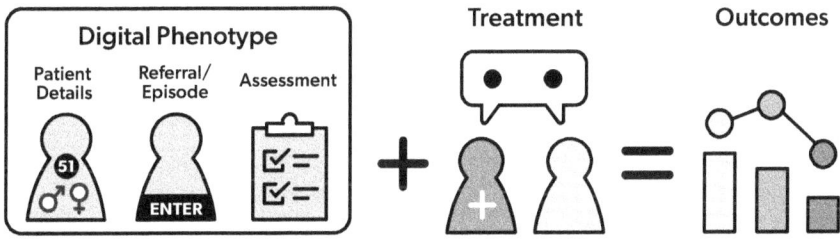

In essence, for every patient we are asking what kind of patient this is, and what therefore the best treatment pathway for them to follow to achieve the best possible outcome would be. It is so simple, in fact, that you might wonder why we are not already doing this, literally anywhere, in the world right now. But as always, the devil is in the detail and I will explore some of the immediate challenges to achieving this vision in more depth as I delve into Themes 1 and 2 in the following chapter. But for now, suffice it to say, the problems are threefold:

1. We have not done enough to standardise the data we collect (coming up next).
2. We do not measure **outcomes** (Theme 1).
3. Our **treatment pathways** are rarely **protocolised** (Theme 2).

To adopt this brave new world, there is much to be done. But the technology is there; we just need to organise ourselves to use it properly.

Standardise to personalise

From one perspective, data-driven healthcare is what results from a fusion of individual care with population health management. At the moment, these two aspects of healthcare have been largely separated in most economies and are often the responsibility of completely different organisations. This naturally works against the two ever coming together, but right now there is a bigger issue to address. In one forum of clinicians, I carelessly used the term 'data-centred healthcare' and instantly regretted it. 'We don't deliver "data-centred" healthcare – we deliver "patient-centred" healthcare,' I was quickly told. On that occasion, referring to Amazon as an example of excellent customer-centred care using a data-centred approach simply made matters worse. Everyone uses it but no one is completely comfortable with what it stands for. There is still something impersonal – and therefore distasteful – about interacting with a huge, data-driven machine, even while receiving the best customer experience from it.

Clinicians, understandably, want to treat everyone as a unique individual and deliver personalised care. In reality, however, each patient's journey is far from unique in its essential elements. Many routine procedures have protocols that are followed by everyone no matter who you are or where you've come from. The sense that your care is personalised is often an illusion. Yes, there may be tweaks here and there but the care you receive will usually be the same as for everyone else. Yet as soon as we start to talk about that care being steered in any shape or form by the vast ocean of data we have previously collected, there's a sense in which the whole thing starts to feel like a huge sausage machine churning out healthy patients from sick ones with all the personalisation stripped out. This isn't the case and misses the point, notwithstanding that patients might anyway prefer a better outcome than a personalised experience, if that really was the choice.

But that isn't the choice. Data-driven approaches, operating at scale, offer the possibility of the most personalised – and therefore personal – healthcare experience yet. Ultimately, the care you receive using these techniques will be based not just on a handful of data points that combine your demographic and diagnostic data, but also your DNA profile and the composition of your microbiome. It will be so personalised that it will truly be unique to you, right down to the precise dose of whatever drug you might end up being prescribed.

To personalise care using data-led techniques, we need to standardise the data. It may seem counterintuitive but the more data we can standardise the more we can personalise the care we deliver. I think it is generally understood that most data items need to be codified in order to be any use at all for any form of processing or analytics. For that reason, the data we collect is often restricted in format (such as dates, postcodes or phone numbers) or limited to selections from drop-down menus (eg gender, ethnicity). Beyond these basic data items, though, we create a vast landscape of free text, often full of spelling mistakes, that is almost impossible to analyse sensibly in a way that can be put to good use. The science of actually doing this – known as natural language processing (NLP) – is advancing rapidly but is still far from being able to drive care in the right direction.

'Standardise to personalise' is the mantra of my vision of

data-driven healthcare. The more data we can standardise, the better. This doesn't stop us from using free text where appropriate but it is always better to combine this with a tick box if we can. For example, I have seen so many questionnaires asking patients to describe their drinking habits using an open question such as 'How much alcohol do you consume in a typical week?' – followed by a free-text box for the answer. If we wanted to know the average weekly alcohol consumption of the patients presenting to us this year compared with last year (and we might – the Covid pandemic saw a sharp rise in alcohol consumption during lockdown that may, or may not, have impacted on mental health referrals), then mountains of free-text responses are not going to give us the answer easily. Far better to front the free-text box with a selection box banding units of alcohol consumed before giving them free rein to describe their week of partying. Even better would be to provide a calculator that does the job of calculating units for them by counting glasses of wine, pints of beer, shorts, etc. Note that I am not advocating abolishing or replacing free-text boxes. They are still important for all sorts of reasons, but wherever possible they should be accompanied by some form of standardised response.

When we talk about standardising data, we are not just referring to the digital phenotype data that describes a patient at the start of their journey. We are talking about standardising everything, including all the events that happen and the outcomes that are achieved. Basically everything that makes up the components in the equation illustrated above. In the next two chapters, I will explore this in the context of outcomes (Theme 1) and treatment pathways (Theme 2).

The digital healthcare record

In the generic sense, patient management systems are described using different terminology around the world. Most common today are the electronic health record or electronic patient record, the emergence of which I described in the previous chapter, that power most hospitals and community services. Still, their definition is evolving and, at the time of writing, EHR/EPR advocates are attempting to restrict these terms specifically to refer to large, integrated systems covering a whole population's hospital and community healthcare needs, with modules for inpatient bed management, outpatients, radiology, pathology, order management, theatres, maternity, therapies, allied health services and community support services, all integrated together with primary care. A system that performs only some of these functions, but not all of them, will not be able to call itself an EHR/EPR and will instead need to find another descriptor.

(As an aside, I am not a fan of this approach. The debate between commissioning monolithic systems that do everything and purchasing best-of-breed for each clinical function has been raging for decades. Thirty years ago, when I first entered the arena of healthcare IT, I came down firmly on favouring the joined-up best-of-breed strategy over the large, multifunctional system that keeps the patient record together and does everything but does it poorly. If anything, technological advances, particularly over the past decade, have swung the argument even further toward a best-of-breed strategy because it is now easier than ever to get systems to talk to each other and build a holistic patient record, removing the main advantage that the monolithic systems had. But this is just a personal view and I understand both sides of the argument, which I suspect will continue for some years to come. I will revisit this particular issue in Theme 5.)

At this point, therefore, I wish to claim a descriptor: the digital healthcare record (DHR). No doubt the phrase digital healthcare record has been bandied about in all sorts of contexts and to mean many different things, but I would like it to refer to something quite specific, namely that a DHR is a system that supports a patient through a healthcare journey, from initial referral to discharge, harnessing the power of digital and data-driven techniques at every step to seek a positive outcome, and most importantly, records those outcomes and learns from them. In the clinical setting in which it is deployed, it will be best-of-breed in that setting because its entire purpose will be to drive positive outcomes for patients with specific but common conditions. So, whether used to support patients with diabetes, musculoskeletal problems, drug and alcohol issues or common mental health disorders, a DHR would be trained to maximise outcomes for each condition.

A DHR is not an EHR but would be able to integrate with it so that important patient data is not lost to the wider healthcare environment. In fact, it would be possible for a population-wide EHR to be supported by several purpose-driven DHRs as part of a local ecosystem of healthcare provision. Importantly, while an EHR is designed to hold comprehensive holistic records for a local population, a DHR would not necessarily be restricted by geography. Being more condition and data focused would enable it to draw on treatments and outcomes from a far wider population base. Indeed, the bigger the population a DHR covers, the better as it would have access to far more data to drive positive outcomes.

A DHR itself may form the centre of its own ecosystem, combining the skills and talents of multiple providers or even apps in the pursuit of offering choice and optimising care pathways for outcome improvement. This system architecture would essentially double down on the best-of-breed strategy by recognising not only that an EHR can be enhanced with condition-specific DHRs, but that DHRs themselves can host care pathways that include other best-of-breed services that may be human or technology based. Essentially, DHRs are the building blocks of a hierarchy of data systems that connect the EHR/EPR at the centre to all the peripheral services and data stores that together make up the whole patient journey.

Note that the DHR would not be the digital *health* record, which would by implication be a wider-ranging set of data capturing everything to do with health and wellbeing. In theory, it would be possible to have a digital *health* record without having any *healthcare* intervention at all, but would use the same data-driven techniques to help individuals maintain and improve fitness and wellbeing by nudging lifestyle changes based on the behaviours and consequences of a broader population. The difference between 'health' and 'healthcare' is important here but the confusion is set to persist as long as EHRs refer to electronic health records and not electronic healthcare records, which is what they really are.

*

In the following chapter, I will explore six themes which I believe will be key to the evolution of the digital healthcare record in the coming years. Not for economic or commercial reasons, primarily, but simply because we (clinicians, managers, IT and data professionals, and suppliers) want to do healthcare right. The absence of a data-led approach at this point in the 21st century, with all the computing power, tools and analytic techniques at our disposal, challenges us as to how much we really want to do our very best for the individual patients in our healthcare services.

8 Key themes

Ultimately, there will be many different facets to achieving the vision for data-driven healthcare, but I believe there are six, specifically, that will require special attention.

Theme 1: Outcomes

The outcomes illusion

A healthcare intervention involves taking a patient on a journey from a place where they are suffering to a place where they have recovered, or at least suffering less. The whole point of embarking on an episode of healthcare is to achieve some sort of outcome; otherwise why do it in the first place? And if a positive outcome is the goal, then surely measuring and recording whether that outcome has been achieved is of paramount importance?

People invariably do a double take when I comment that healthcare services across the world rarely or never monitor outcomes. Intuitively that can't be right, can it? Surely we know whether we are doing patients any good or not? Well yes – and no. Almost all healthcare IT systems will record whether you leave an episode of care alive or dead. So that's a start. But other than that, everything that gets recorded is really an input and the outcome is assumed. For example, if a patient has a hip replacement, that is recorded and referred to as if it is an outcome. But it isn't really. It confirms that a patient has had a new hip put into them; it doesn't confirm that they are now able to walk freely and without pain. That bit – the real healthcare outcome – is rarely recorded, or if it is, it is buried in some free-text, follow-up outpatient note where it is of little use to anyone.

Regardless of whether services are trying to be data-driven or not, outcomes should be recorded much more than they are. It's an essential element of our healthcare systems that is missing: the part that tells us whether the journey we've been on has had a happy ending or not. It is assumed that a patient who has been discharged and doesn't come back means that everything is hunky dory. And mostly it is, but that is a bold assumption to make and hunky dory is not exactly scientifically robust as a measure of outcome. Across the world, healthcare records tell the stories of patients on journeys with the last chapter missing.

The lack of routine outcome data is bad enough but even worse is when a patient does return with a problem, indicating that they haven't had a good outcome. Patient records are notoriously patchy in terms of data quality and completeness but outpatient records are generally far worse than inpatient records. So, while a relatively complete inpatient record – fully coded – might give the impression that all of these inputs have led to positive outcomes, the incomplete and poorly codified follow-up outpatient record might have told a very different story.

The consequences of not measuring outcomes

Major healthcare scandals seem to appear at the rate of around two per year, at least those that make the national headlines. When a problem does surface, I am always amazed by how long the problem has been going on – and consequently how many patients have been adversely affected – before it was picked up. And even then, rarely is it a revelation provided by the data. Usually it's through an individual or group of patients, or a member of staff turned whistleblower. This is the dark side of not recording outcomes.

Consider the scandals in the maternity units at Royal Shrewsbury, Morecambe Bay or Nottingham, similarly at Mid Staffordshire Hospitals, Bristol Children's Hospital heart unit, the gynaecology surgical mesh debacle or even rogue individuals such as Harold Shipman. A whole book could be written on each of these, but they all had one feature in common. The issues were prolonged in part either because outcome data didn't exist or because it wasn't being looked at.

While we primarily want to use outcomes to improve patient care and create a positive feedback cycle, the absence of outcome monitoring can have dire consequences, not only affecting individual patients and clinicians, but also undermining the whole healthcare system. If outcomes were recorded and monitored systematically, it is highly likely that hundreds and thousands of patients would have avoided being harmed. Yet despite repeated scandals with this common underlying theme, outcomes are still not recorded as a matter of course. In fact, many IT systems designed to manage patient care do not even have room for them.

Black box thinking

In his book *Black Box Thinking* (2015), Matthew Syed contrasts the attitude of the medical profession with that of the airline industry, and it is well worth a read. After every air crash, everything is exposed and made transparent in order to discover the root cause of the crash, learn the lessons and ensure that such an accident never happens again. This has been happening for decades, with the result that 2017 was hailed as the first year that no plane crashed – and consequently no one died in an air accident – anywhere in the world. Pilots, in particular, welcome this openness and are encouraged to be transparent about their own mistakes. They do so for three reasons. First, they are invested; if the plane goes down, then they go down with it. Second, it is understood that the lessons learned may save their lives and the lives of their colleagues in the future. Third, to achieve this level of openness, the airline industry has adopted a no-blame culture that does not penalise mistakes, instead valuing learning the lessons and subsequent prevention over attributing responsibility and accountability.

In contrast, clinicians do not suffer with their patients, and the accountability and medico-legal cultures that have been allowed to evolve in healthcare work directly against a spirit of openness, to the detriment of both the professions and the patients. In short, clinicians are not incentivised to measure outcomes and indeed the opposite is often true as clinicians might see outcome measurement as simply an evidence base to be used to point out their failings, possibly with career-limiting consequences. The consequence of this omission is that there are clinicians practising today who cannot provide any evidence that they have benefited even one single patient through their interventions, even though their outcomes might be extraordinarily positive and their clinical practice would provide exceptional opportunities for others to learn.

Positive feedback

While the measurement of outcomes is seen by many clinicians as a stick to beat them with when they fail to perform to an expected standard, I consider this perspective can only be viewed as a failure of the whole healthcare system. To apportion blame should be the last reason why outcomes are measured. The real benefit of outcome monitoring is to use the data as part of a culture of continuous improvement. Positive outcomes beget even more positive outcomes. Negative outcomes should encourage understanding, learning, sharing, greater collaboration and perhaps more training and development, all leading to more positive outcomes in the future. Against these benefits, hiding problems and apportioning blame are poor relations.

Data-driven healthcare – and all the potential it brings – cannot work if we do not measure outcomes. Why? Because its primary purpose is to improve outcomes so it ceases to exist as a logical possibility if outcomes aren't measured. We need the feedback from those outcomes in the past to benefit the patients of the future. A digital healthcare record – as defined earlier – ultimately has its raison d'être in improved outcomes for patients, otherwise it is just another patient-management system collecting inputs and spewing out bills and performance statistics based on resources consumed. Whether or not system architecture evolves in the way I envisioned in the last chapter, the expansion of outcome measurement has to be a major theme in healthcare service design and IT development over the coming years. If it isn't, then we will never do healthcare properly.

Theme 2: Care pathways

Protocolised care

While there are circumstances where all that can be achieved for a patient is to maintain their current level of health or manage a decline, in most cases healthcare is about taking a patient on a journey to a place of better health.

In an ideal world, every patient would be treated as a unique individual whose particular circumstances at that time in some way warrants special treatment. This does not mean every patient is selfish and wants more than other patients, such as more time with the doctor, more tests, more drugs. Often it can mean a patient wants less – but quicker – attention. They know what is wrong with them, they know what they need to sort out the problem, they just want to cut through the red tape, arrive at the front of the queue and get the treatment they know works as quickly and as painlessly as the system permits, without affecting anyone else and consuming as few resources as possible.

Similarly, every clinician wants to treat each patient as an individual, a unique case who may have similarities to other patients but whose particular life journey differs to a greater or lesser degree from their peers and needs to be taken into account. All patients are autonomous human beings and should be treated as such, given as much time as they need and an individual care plan to suit their circumstances.

That's in an ideal world. It is not the one we live in.

Given this very human perspective, shared by clinicians and patients alike, it is not surprising that the word 'protocolisation' causes a negative reaction in all stakeholders in the healthcare system. It is not even a pleasant-sounding word. Say it to yourself. Does it sound like something you want to have happen to you? Exactly. No one wants to feel as if they are on some kind of production line or in a sausage machine. The very idea smacks of the opposite of care and is something that should have no place in the healthcare system.

Yet I would like to argue that protocolised care is not only what the health system needs more of, but is, in this new era of data and digital, the route to achieving the personalised and effective care everyone desires.

Everyday protocolisation

In fact, in this sense, every day people unwittingly allow themselves to be protocolised in order to receive a personalised service. When you load your social media feeds – whether Facebook, X, Instagram or LinkedIn, you receive a page of information that is unique to you. Yet the software that loads the page – the protocols driving the system – are exactly the same for everybody. Just because you have logged in, the Facebook servers do not run a different program with your name on it. The code that runs is universal. What is different is the data. When you go to your Amazon home page, the same thing happens. The same code runs but the product recommendations will be unique to you, based on your history and those whose shopping habits are similar to yours. Ask your best friend to recommend a book for you to read and they may or may not select something you will like. Ask Amazon the same question and, without knowing you at all in any personal capacity, the chance that it will select a book you will enjoy is much higher.

All these online services – and many others like them – have been hugely successful because they personalise the content they serve to each individual user. They can do this because they have protocolised every aspect of their virtual ecosystems. Everyone gets the same service. Everyone gets a personal service. It sounds contradictory but it is happening every second of every single day all around the world. It is an extremely powerful yet simple principle that has made billionaires of the pioneers of these applications in only a few years.

So, the big question is: how can this principle be leveraged in healthcare?

Introducing the care pathway record

In a healthcare setting, conceptually there are really only two things you need to standardise to put this principle into motion: the data that is collected and the route map showing the various pathways that patients could follow as they navigate the healthcare system. While I have already explored the argument for data standardisation in the previous chapter, here I will be looking more closely at the latter element: the route map.

Let me first of all explore the difference between a care plan and a care pathway. Today, these two terms are often used interchangeably but there are subtle yet important differences between them and it will be particularly important to understand the meaning of the term 'care pathway' as I proceed through the chapter, as this term is the much friendlier-sounding version of 'protocolised care' that I referred to earlier.

Care plans

A 'care plan' – often called an 'individualised care plan' – in its fundamental form is a document that lists a patient's *individual* care needs and selected treatment options as they proceed through a particular healthcare system. It lists, in sequential order, assessments, diagnoses and the services a patient will receive, by whom and at what time. Often they will be based around set goals with a timeline or set of interim stages to achieve those goals. They can take many different forms but an example of a simple care plan is shown overleaf.

Though often based on standard templates, each care plan has the potential to be unique to each individual patient. They are most often used by the nursing professions and often altered daily as the needs of the patient evolve during treatment. For this reason, a care plan may be stored electronically or on paper. Often it is created electronically but then printed out and altered manually.

Patient Care Plan: Type 2 Diabetes Mellitus

Name: Jane Doe
Associated conditions: hypertension and mild obesity

Overall Goal

To effectively manage blood sugar and blood pressure levels, reduce body weight by 5%, and improve overall quality of life through lifestyle modifications and consistent medical management.

Weekly Action Plan

Week	Primary Goal	Key Actions
Week 1	Establish foundational habits and monitoring.	• Start monitoring blood glucose daily and blood pressure three times per week. • Set up a weekly pillbox to ensure proper medication adherence. • Begin incorporating 15 minutes of daily stress-management techniques.
Week 2	Integrate physical activity and initial dietary changes.	• Begin at least 30 minutes of moderate-intensity aerobic exercise five days per week. • Start working with a registered dietitian to create a personalised meal plan. • Begin tracking your weight weekly to establish a baseline.
Week 3	Refine diet and build on exercise habits.	• Begin following the personalised meal plan focusing on whole foods and non-starchy vegetables. • Incorporate light strength training twice a week. • Record your blood glucose levels before and two hours after your main meals.
Week 4	Ensure consistency and seek support.	• Adhere strictly to the prescribed medication schedule. • Participate in a local diabetes support group or an online health education seminar. • Review your weekly progress with your doctor if necessary.
Week 5 & Beyond	Maintain and plan for the future.	• Continue all daily and weekly actions consistently. • Attend all scheduled follow-up appointments with your primary care doctor. • Schedule your annual visits with the ophthalmologist and podiatrist.

Contingency Plan

- **Hypoglycemia (low blood sugar):** If blood sugar drops below 70 mg/dL, consume 15 grams of a fast-acting carbohydrate (eg, glucose tablet, 1⁄8 oz of fruit juice).
- **Hyperglycemia (high blood sugar):** If blood sugar is consistently high (over 180 mg/dL for two consecutive readings), the patient will contact their physician immediately.

Care pathways

A care pathway operates more at the system level, setting out the various routes that a patient could follow as they progress through the system. It has the appearance of a flow chart with entry points, decision points and exit options interspersed between a range of diagnostic and treatment stages. Care pathways are planned or possible patient journeys for all patients based on clinical protocols and not usually for an individual patient. Here is a simple example.

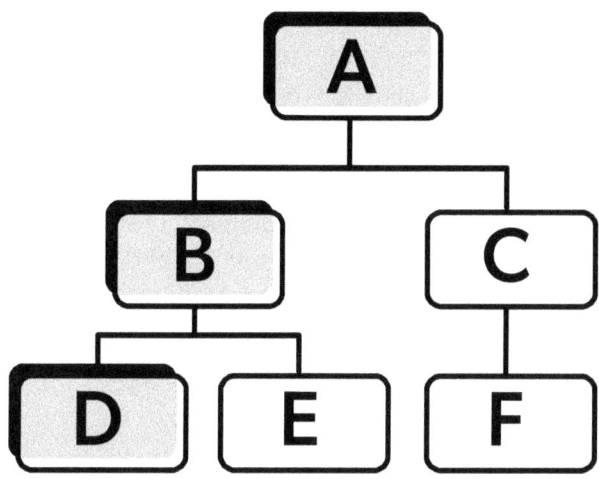

The route a patient takes through the care pathway is known as their individual *care pathway record*, sometimes referred to as a patient journey map, and highlighted in bold in the example. It is no longer a plan but an actual record of the patient journey during and after an episode of care. A patient's individual pathway record is not necessarily unique to that patient. It is perfectly possible for a patient to trace a route through the care pathway that no previous patient has followed; however, it is more likely that a patient will follow a pathway that has been followed many times before. There are invariably far more patients than routes through the care pathway but some of these routes may be so rare that very few patients follow them.

Unlike a care plan, which is primarily sequential, care pathways can loop patients back to a place they've been before in order to try a different route. This would normally result in the abandonment of the previous care plan and the creation of a new one.

In the same ideal world referred to before (which doesn't exist), for each clinical condition the care pathway would be globally universal. But that isn't realistic or practicable. Pragmatically, the care pathway needs to reflect the regimes and options that are available on the ground locally, with different entry points, the range of diagnostic tests on offer, decision points based on local protocols and the range of treatment options available in the local health system. Within this local setting, however, the care pathway should be the same and navigated by all patients.

This does not mean that the care pathway cannot change. In fact, as you will see, the whole point of adopting this approach is to make enhancements to the pathway over time to effect positive and gradual improvements in patient outcomes and operational efficiency. We naturally need to allow for the possibility of new entry points, the addition of new diagnostic tests or treatment regimes, and for the potential onward referral of patients to new services that emerge over time. Similarly, we may move some tests or treatments from the care pathway that are no longer considered to be effective or cost efficient.

Benefiting from care pathway data

Standardised care pathways serve two primary functions. First, they can provide a kind of macro checklist ensuring that every patient gets treated to the same standard, is given the same options and that nothing important is omitted from consideration, even if it is not ultimately taken up. The power of checklists in healthcare cannot be underestimated. Checklists were first introduced in the 1930s in the aviation industry in response to the increasing complexity pilots were experiencing in the cockpit. As more instrumentation and controls were added, it became more likely that mistakes would be made. And they were, sometimes with devastating consequences. Similarly, in the operating theatre, new surgical advances have appeared at an extraordinary rate over the past few decades, but this has also brought about increasing complexity and a higher likelihood that complications might arise. According to the World Health Organization, which introduced recommended surgical checklists in 2008, mistakes in theatres around the world were causing injuries resulting in new disabilities to seven million people every year (WHO 2008).

In 2009, *The Checklist Manifesto*, by Atul Gawande, became an international bestseller and heralded a revolution in operating theatre procedures. Early studies have shown that deaths resulting from surgical errors fell by one third in the immediate aftermath of the introduction of checklists. In the same way, standardised care pathways can ensure that patients are only able to navigate safe routes through the healthcare system and that important steps are not forgotten.

The second – and in the context of data-driven healthcare the most important – reason for standardising a care pathway is to collect consistent data that allows the care pathway journeys to be analysed and improved. While care pathways – in the form of a protocolised plan for a healthcare journey – are becoming quite commonplace, care pathway *records* are not. This widespread adoption of care pathway records is therefore the primary thing that needs to change.

Significant intelligence can be derived from a care pathway record containing even the most basic data collection such as in the example shown, where only the date and time the patient reaches each stage of the pathway is collected.

Step	Stage	Date / Time	Days in stage
1	Referral received	2 Jan 2025 10:12	1
2	Check eligibility	3 Jan 2025 14:03	0
3	Enter waitlist for assessment	3 Jan 2025 14:24	10
4	Triage assessment	13 Jan 2025 14:00	0
5	Enter group therapy waitlist	13 Jan 2025 15:14	21
6	Begin group therapy	3 Feb 2025 10:00	41
7	Review progress	16 Mar 2025 13:20	0
8	Begin individual CBT sessions	16 Mar 2025 14:10	44
9	Review progress	30 April 2025 09:30	0
10	Discharge	30 April 2025 10:37	0

Here the data in each row is simply time-stamping the moves as patients step from one part of the care pathway (ie move along the flow chart) to the next, recording where the patient went and for how long. This simple data set alone provides the potential to undertake a range of analyses and logistical improvements.

Identifying popular routes

Some routes through the care pathway will inevitably be more popular than others, and in many cases this might result in a significant proportion of patients following these favoured routes. Across a wide range of health services, it would not be unusual for 80 per cent of patients to follow the most common route, leaving the remaining 20 per cent following alternatives (some of which may be only slight deviations from the most popular route).

An analysis of the most popular routes taken through a care pathway with 16 different stages might look as follows:

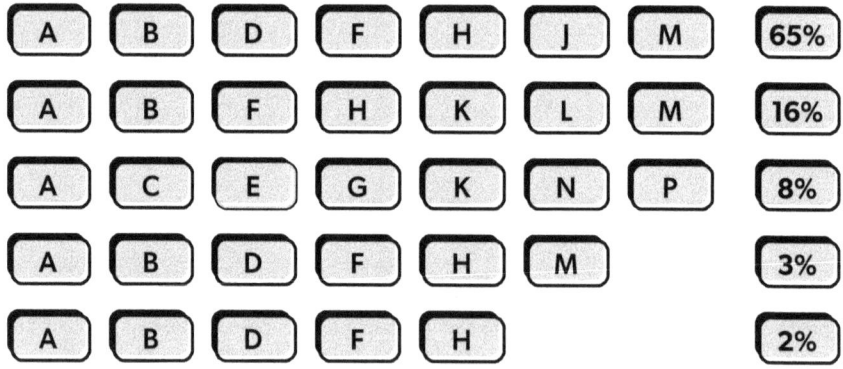

The most popular route through the pathway is A>B>D>F>H>J>M, which is taken by 65 per cent (almost two thirds) of the total. If we want to make the biggest impact as soon as possible, it therefore makes sense to focus our attention on this popular route and make it as effective and efficient as possible because that will reap the biggest benefits for both patients and staff. Having streamlined and optimised this route as far as possible, we would then move on to the next most popular route (in this case representing 16 per cent of patient journeys) and repeat.

Note, however, that the second most popular route (A>B>F>H>K>L>M) shares the first two stages (A>B) with the most popular route. So it makes sense to focus our attention on these first as that will actually benefit 81 per cent of patients. In reality, these are likely to be the procedures that take place around referral, initial assessment and triage, which will be common for most patients. Only when we have gathered basic information about a patient will we begin to have the data required to start making differential decisions about care pathways (or draw up individual care plans). Not surprisingly, many of the processes a patient experiences near the entrance to a healthcare system are administrative and these are often the easiest to automate and optimise.

Today, at most airports, you will check in for your flights and register your bags using a screen. Similarly, at McDonald's, you now order your burger and fries in the same way – without any human contact. These processes have been automated first because they are the same for everyone, so that's what makes the most sense to prioritise. It will not be long before you are welcomed at the hospital door by a virtual concierge who will deal with all the admin before alerting the doctor that you have arrived, while displaying a map telling you how to find the appropriate department. In a large hospital, with a maze of corridors, this map will already have been sent to your mobile phone so you don't have to memorise it. After all, how many appointments have been missed because the patient has got lost in the building?

The key point here is that to improve the system we first need to examine the system and see how it is being used. Standardising the care pathways, collecting simple data (automatically) and analysing it simply to tell us what to work on first is a good start.

Analyse decision points

At any stage that a patient enters in a care pathway, there could be more than one exit. In order to determine where a patient goes next, a decision has to be made. These decisions can be automated or determined by human beings, who could in theory be the clinician or clinicians treating the patient, or the patients themselves.

Decisions may be:

- rule-based (eg this patient is not funded so should not be allowed to go further; this patient has an allergy that prevents certain options for treatment)
- threshold-based (eg this patient has a depression score above X so needs to follow the pathway for severe depression)
- clinician-based (eg based on my many years of experience of seeing symptoms like this I think you might actually have a heart condition and we should refer you down the cardiac assessment pathway)
- risk-based (eg given your genetic profile and family history of cervical cancer, more regular smear tests are advised)
- patient-based (eg given the choice I'd prefer to have a dental implant rather than a bridge)
- a blend of some or all of the above.

What protocols are in place will have a bearing on the decisions being made and these decisions will have an impact on the rest of the care pathway. For example, sending too many patients through one exit may swamp resources in that part of the care pathway and prompt a different decision to be made for future patients. This might result from changing a rule, moving a threshold or by the patient or clinician making a different decision. Having the historical data available allows us to model what the impact of making a different decision might be. In the case of the patient with severe depression, we might decide to try lifting the depression score threshold to (X+1) and introduce another pathway for patients with a score of X. What might this look like? It could simply involve the introduction of a new member of staff who can offer a particular kind of therapy to patients with a score up to X but not above X, thereby alleviating the pressure on those clinicians working at the intensive end.

Sometimes, some interesting insights might be gained from analysing those decision points where there is an active choice being made (ie by a human). Consider the following example.

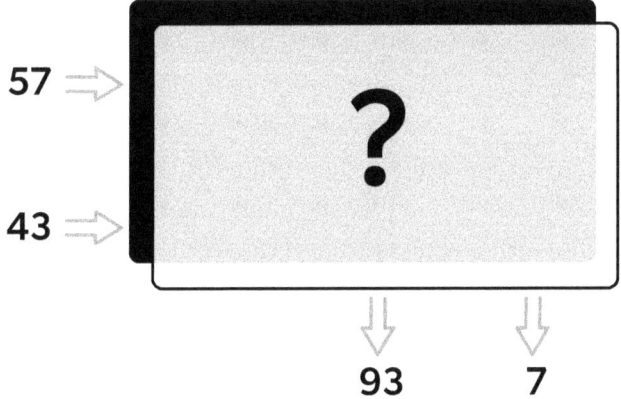

In this example, 100 patients are entering a care pathway stage through two entrances, with 57 patients coming from one direction and 43 from the other. Let us assume that this stage involves a clinical review and a decision needs to be made whether to send a patient out of one of two exits (left or right) in order to follow the next appropriate stage of the care pathway. In this case the decision is being made to exit 93 patients down the left-hand branch of the pathway with only 7 patients following the right-hand branch.

This in itself might be interesting to explore. Why are only 7 per cent of patients being sent to the right? Is the right-hand branch necessary? Does it improve outcomes for those patients? Is it a cost-effective use of resources? But things can become even more interesting when we superimpose the decision maker onto the analysis:

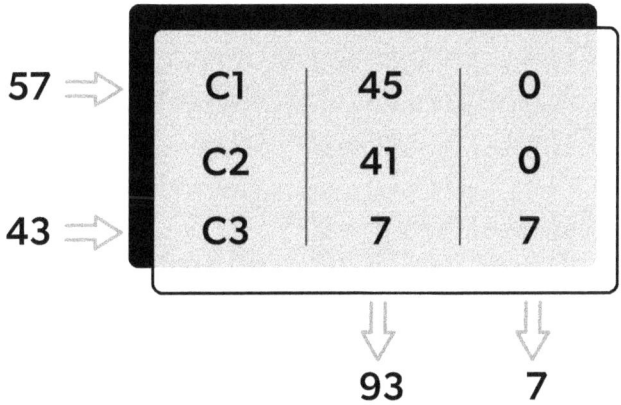

Now we find that three clinicians (C1, C2, C3) are involved in making these decisions and two of them are sending all of their patients to the left. Only clinician C is using the right-hand care pathway and they are using it for half of their patients. Of course, this might be entirely appropriate depending on who the clinician is, what knowledge and skills they have, which patients they are seeing, etc. But the question may also give rise to some interesting answers that prompt a change in the decision-making protocol if those answers are not considered to be befitting the circumstances.

Measuring journey times

What happens between stages in the care pathway can be just as important as what happens in them. Patient journeys that are not efficient can exacerbate problems and patients can deteriorate – sometimes quite rapidly – while waiting for the next intervention to commence.

Using a care pathway approach – where every move between stages is automatically date and time stamped – we can measure the journey times between any two stages. This might include from *referral to first assessment*, which is effectively the waiting time to be seen by a specialist. Equally we might want to measure *referral to discharge*, indicating the total journey time for a patient to travel through the system. Or it might be *assessment to first intervention*, which exposes another waiting list – and consequent delays – after the first wait for the initial assessment.

In fact, depending on the clinical service, there might be reasons why we want to measure journey times from any one point in the care pathway to any other point, all of which could potentially provide a wealth of information to support workflow improvements.

Identifying bottlenecks

An analysis of staged journey times, as described above, and/or an analysis of the number of patients in each stage of the care pathway, can be used to identify bottlenecks. These can often be ironed out quite effectively by redeploying resources to achieve a better balance and flow. In many senses, this is no different to optimising a production line to ensure product doesn't build up at any one point and the manufacturing industry has established ways to achieve this over many decades.

Rationalising pathways

An analysis of what is really happening during a patient's journey will often show that there are many pathways being followed that are all quite similar. Combining them together and agreeing a common protocol that doesn't compromise patient care can both reduce complexity and help streamline workflows, improving efficiency.

Pathway optimisation

In conclusion, simply by recording the date and time that patients move through the different stages of their journey, data that can be captured easily and without any manual data input, a whole world opens up that can lead to substantial improvements in both efficiency and outcomes. All of the analyses described above can be derived from that simple foundation. And those analyses can be combined in all sorts of ways to help identify improvements that can be made to care pathway journeys to benefit both clinicians and patients.

Combining care pathways and outcome data

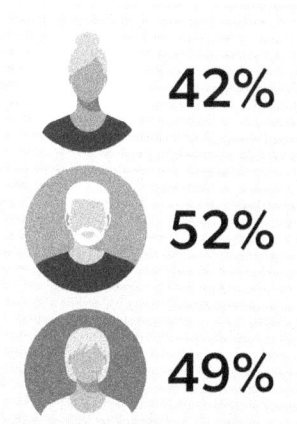

It is important to recognise that optimising a care pathway does not mean reducing it to a one-size-fits-all sausage machine, and this is perhaps where patient care pathways differ from production lines. There may be reasons why different cohorts of patients require different pathways and this might most easily be exposed in the outcome data.

Take the example shown here (left) where three patient cohorts – ie people with similar digital phenotypes (profiles) to Alice, Bob and Charlie – have achieved average outcome scores (out of 100) as shown.

At face value, it would appear that people like Bob are achieving better outcomes than Alice and Charlie.

Now look what happens when we take our simple care pathway and look at the outcomes achieved using different routes.

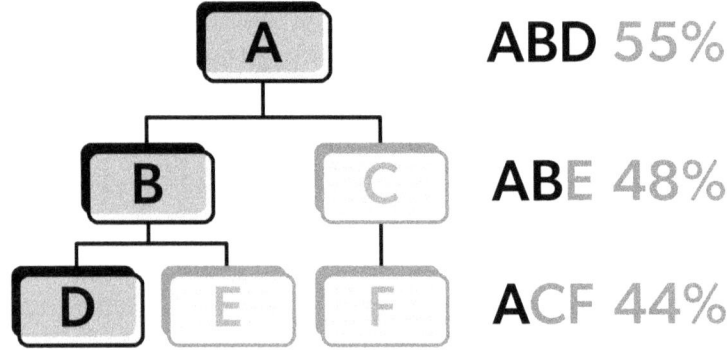

Again, it would appear that patients using route A>B>D do better in terms of outcome scores. However, if we combine the cohort outcome data together with the pathway outcome data, we might see an analysis like this:

		ABD	ABE	ACF
	42%	48%	36%	40%
	52%	50%	54%	48%
	49%	47%	46%	60%
		55%	48%	44%

Here we see that Alice, and patients like her, would indeed do significantly better if they followed the pathway (A>B>D) that was shown overall to produce the best outcomes. However, Bob, and patients like him, who achieved the highest overall outcome score (52) could do marginally better (54) if they were all to follow route A>B>E through the care pathway, even though pathway A>B>D has been shown to achieve the best outcomes overall. Most tellingly, the pathway with the worst outcomes overall (A>C>F) would actually benefit Charlie and her cohort most of all, enabling them to push their outcome score up from an average of 49 to 60.

Combining care pathway and outcome data in this way has the potential to unleash enormous benefits for a wide range of healthcare services. This is the essence of data-driven healthcare.

Theme 3: Decision support

Data in, nothing out

If, historically, healthcare IT has been regarded as an almost universally hated industry, in my experience the primary reason for that is that almost all systems were designed with the sole purpose of sucking data in – and sometimes not very efficiently – but then not giving anything back. In the NHS, any insights obtained from the data are often only available at national level through the collection of minimum datasets. Trust boards often report flying blind when it comes to activity performance metrics. Front-line clinicians, though, could be forgiven for perceiving their systems as black holes as they pour data into various forms and fields while subsequently receiving little if any benefit from all that effort.

For IT suppliers, there are two responses to this: provide ready access to the data so that customers can build their own data analytics teams and do whatever they want; or build analytics modules into the software. Increasingly, healthcare IT companies are adopting the former over the latter. There are lots of good reasons why they are opting to take this approach. For one thing, it means they don't have to invest in developing the analytical tools, which can be notoriously complex and tricky. It keeps prices down and pushes the problem on to the customer to solve. Customers, in turn, welcome the power and control this gives them but often don't appreciate that the total cost of ownership of the IT system is much higher. But the bigger issue with this approach is that it still doesn't give clinicians on the front line an easy way of surfacing insights from the data. And usually, the clinicians at the coal face are last in line to be able to access resource from their analytics team. The consequence of this, of course, is that data quality deteriorates. If you don't get anything out of a system, why spend the time and effort assuring the quality of what you put in?

Analytics for everyone

In this day and age, access to analytics should be ubiquitous. We should no longer accept a situation where data insights are only available to the chosen few or those with the skills to surface them. This doesn't mean that system suppliers need to reinvent the wheel and create bespoke modules at great expense. The state of the art today includes a wide array of powerful business intelligence platforms that can be integrated or embedded into software for all to use rather than just being the domain of the data analytics team. And this doesn't even mean that system users need to develop the technical skills themselves. It is now possible to provide a vast array of configurable, high-quality, visually stunning dashboards that even avid technophobes can get to grips with.

The benefits of providing analytics to everyone cannot be understated. It gives individual clinicians and clinical teams the power to manage their own affairs and to introduce a culture of continuous improvement internally without having to rely on external resources that may not be available to them, or who may not really have the clinical domain knowledge to analyse the data appropriately, even if they do have the technical skills. And, of course, if clinicians are able to access the insights directly they will be much more concerned to achieve higher levels of quality and completeness.

Theme 4: Workflow

Is the tail wagging the dog?

One of the most frequent complaints about healthcare IT is that the way the system works isn't the way clinicians work. This can often result in clinicians having to change their work practices to something that is at best less than optimal and sometimes inappropriate. There are a number of reasons for this.

In the early days, the development of IT systems was purely in the domain of geeks whose structured, logical thinking – and lack of clinical domain knowledge – didn't reflect the real world. This has gradually changed over the past few decades. Software developers are not all computer scientists – far from it – and today originate from a wide variety of backgrounds. Moreover, the past 15 years has also seen the emergence of the user experience (UX) role, which was created to bridge the gap between front-line users and back-end developers. In highly customer-led organisations it is the UX team that leads the development cycle, ensuring that front-line users have interfaces that they can relate to and which mirror their daily lives. Software teams have equally divided into front-end and back-end developers, the former ensuring that the actual user experience works efficiently and reflects the designer's intentions.

Even so, users have not then been properly consulted, or user engagement has been little more than a token gesture. It is not necessary for users themselves to be based in software teams. That can reap obvious benefits but, apart from removing clinicians from care provision, it also poses risks when the embedded users do not adequately reflect the wider user community, driving the software development down a blind alley.

Most of the world's leading patient management systems have foundations built on legacy code that reflected an older clinical regime. Despite attempts to modernise and adjust the code to reflect practice today, often it is not possible to hide the fact that the underlying technical architecture is no longer fit for purpose.

Large monolithic healthcare IT systems often have just one generic workflow that is used by all clinical teams. These are based on the registration > referral > assessment > treatment > discharge model I discussed in Chapter 7, so they largely work. But they do not distinguish between the specific workflow needs of individual clinical teams operating in different specialties and so will always struggle to be best of breed, and often simply to be efficient.

Workflows can vary between clinical teams in different locations, even when operating in the same speciality. This could be because one workflow has evolved to be inefficient, illogical or not reflecting best practice, but has become set in stone. More likely, it is simply because there is more than one way to get the job done, and each is equally effective.

Developing software with strong workflows is challenging. From an individual clinician's point of view, the best software will be focused on their specific role in their specific specialty in their specific context. It is also unrealistic, inefficient and almost always commercially unviable. Software development is a balancing act between the needs of the many and the needs of the few. The trick is to get the needs of the many right while building in enough flexibility to adapt to local requirements.

Note that in Theme 2, the care pathway is not fixed for all time and for all services. It facilitates workflows by reflecting patient journeys, but these can vary from patient to patient and the pathways themselves can evolve, with stages being added and removed as required. Ideally, the system would prompt users in their respective roles to perform actions as patients reach each stage of the pathway. These actions (completing forms, running tests, booking appointments, etc) should be under the control of users and created locally, though there is no reason why default standard workflows couldn't be included. In this way, designed properly, clinical workflows can be made to reflect patient flows through the care pathway, working together in harmony.

In this age of healthcare systems under pressure, with increasing demands on the system, the drive for service efficiency is all important. IT can help enormously in this regard but the systems that emerge as the market leaders will be those that get the workflows right. And this is much more likely to happen with a digital healthcare record solution the focus of which is to be the best of breed in a specific clinical setting.

Theme 5: Interoperability

Imagine this

You are a lead clinician who is offered a new digital health record for your department or specialty. Everything about this system is better than the more generic electronic patient record that your employer has been mandating across the organisation for years. It is designed specifically to support the profile of patients you treat on a daily basis, with an array of bells and whistles to help you provide state-of-the-art care. Its workflows match yours and common tasks such as registering and referring patients, managing their appointments and tracking their progress take half the time that you've been used to experiencing with your current system. It records the data you want to record and much of it is captured as a by-product of your daily clinical practice and not requiring additional tasks on top of your timetabled clinical workload. This new system is programmed with specific assessment and risk tools for your patient cohorts, and alerts are both appropriate and helpful.

Moreover, unlike the system you've been using, which captures little more than whether the patient is alive or dead at the end of their treatment episode, with perhaps a smattering of additional morbidity observations, patient outcomes – the outcomes you're actually seeking from your interventions rather than the inputs you're providing – are monitored and recorded systematically and can be used both to support the care of the individual patient and for wider population analysis to benefit patients in the future.

All in all, this new system allows you to spend more time with each patient and to see many more patients each year, saving you significant time and money while at the same time improving outcomes and providing a platform for continual improvement.

However, there are three immediate snags.

First, in adopting this new system, you would be separating out your portion of the patient record from any other data held about them on the current system. For most patients, this is not really a concern, since their only interaction with your organisation is the one they have with you. However, many others have multiple issues and these can't always or best be treated in isolation. Fragmenting the patient record can introduce inefficiencies and duplication, require clinicians to access multiple systems rather than one and can ultimately lead to accusations that the care being provided is not 'patient centred'.

Second, your new all-singing, all-dancing system isn't free. Though it might save considerably more than it costs, there will be an initial investment required to unlock these savings and it is unlikely that the costs of the current system will be markedly reduced simply because one clinical team is no longer using it.

Third, no IT system comes without some housekeeping and maintenance, but most clinicians and healthcare managers do not want to look after an IT infrastructure and don't have the skills to do so. IT support departments would much rather look after one big EPR system than a myriad of smaller departmental systems, the perception being that it makes their lives easier, only needing to be conversant with one technology.

So, what to do?

The case for interoperability

In healthcare, interoperability refers to the ability of systems to cooperate with other systems in sharing and exchanging data, primarily data containing patient information. Most healthcare services around the world comprise islands of healthcare provision disconnected from the rest of the system, such that the full information about any given patient is fragmented and scattered across a number of platforms. This results in clinicians trying to treat patients with access to only partial information about them, which can have significant implications for outcomes and indeed patient safety.

On the other hand, where healthcare providers have selected systems not on their ability to hold the whole patient record but on their functionality and features for the specific context of their clinical practice, they are at least using systems that are fit for purpose.

This dilemma has been the primary feature of the digital

healthcare landscape for many decades, and the preferred approach has oscillated between a single system versus best-of-breed strategy many times over those years. Interestingly, while some health economies (including countries) pursue one of these two strategies, it is not unusual to find others going in completely the opposite direction.

At the time of writing, the UK is primarily pursuing a one-system-fits-all strategy (albeit not officially), despite much local and supplier resistance. Ironically, this tendency away from best-of-breed systems is happening just as the emergent technology enabling systems to talk properly to each other – facilitating joined-up healthcare between fragmented patient records – has finally arrived!

Building ecosystems

In Chapter 7, where I introduced the concept of the digital healthcare record (DHR), I discussed how data-driven DHRs, focused on supporting care for patients with specific conditions, could form part of a larger healthcare ecosystem. I also rehearsed how the push toward locality-based EHRs was driven by the need for clinicians to have access to all relevant patient data, and that this was most easily achieved by having all of that data in one system.

If there is a place for any flavour of patient management system in the future, its key features will need to include integration with other systems in the wider health (and social) care economy. Too many systems today create silos of healthcare that do not talk to the rest of the system, with detrimental consequences for patients. This should no longer be acceptable. It is only a relatively recent development but technology today (eg APIs) provides the means to create a joined-up healthcare system and it should be embraced. In truth, the very survival of best-of-breed systems depends on prioritising interoperability and getting this right. Complacency is not an option.

The EHR approach is short sighted because, while achieving the aim of keeping all data together, it does so by forcing clinicians to use suboptimal functionality, constraining competition and ultimately stifling innovation. EHRs have their place but the one-size-fits-all approach cannot be permitted to be the only game in town. And equally, EHRs must not be permitted to ignore the wider ecosystem and justify their own monopolistic existence simply by refusing to talk to the other systems within their vicinity.

This points to the biggest challenge for interoperability. In the healthcare IT ecosystem today, some players are incentivised to integrate with other systems while others – primarily the larger systems – are not. Ultimately, all systems that do not do justice to this convergence or interoperability agenda will be driven from the market. But in the meantime, there is an imbalance in incentives, and interoperability between any two systems is only possible where there is willingness on both sides to make it happen. This is best addressed through contracts. Healthcare providers who wish to maintain a mix of best-of-breed alongside their main EHRs have the power to make it happen by mandating each party to cooperate as part of the contracting process.

Theme 6: Patient first

Almost every patient healthcare record system on the planet today has one design philosophy in common: it is used by clinicians to manage patients. Clinical staff own and operate the technology to aid their work albeit ultimately to benefit their patients. But imagine if the EHRs of the future were designed to be more collaborative, with patients and clinicians working on a digital platform together in the dual pursuit of health improvement for both the individual and the service as a whole, each having tailored access to the system to perform operations appropriate to their role in the collaboration. This is already beginning to happen. Today, many patients are able to book appointments, access their own notes and test results, retrieve prescriptions and monitor their own outcomes through patient-facing portals.

But take this concept one step further and imagine a health record owned by the patient, managing their own care and only calling on clinicians as and when they need specialist input. In the not-too-distant future, it is far from inconceivable that patients will be able to self-diagnose, self-medicate and manage their healthcare for a whole range of conditions, using a combination of medically verified assessment data, remote testing and AI-driven knowledge bases. This doesn't remove the role of the clinician (though in many cases it could); however, it allows clinicians to focus on the more complex events, leaving routine cases to manage themselves with only light-touch supervision.

Conceptually, and technically, much of this is possible today. Culturally, it isn't.

Power to the patients

If the digital health revolution ultimately aims to achieve anything, I believe it is about putting more power in the patients' hands, transforming what is currently a patriarchal system into one which is much more collaborative. It is about a shift in the balance of control, from clinician to patient. This doesn't mean that patients have to manage their own health. They can still cede control to clinicians; the point is that it will be their choice.

It cannot be emphasised enough that technology is not really the issue here. The adoption of patient-driven healthcare requires a paradigm shift in perspective, and even the current move towards a more collaborative model is inching forward at a relatively glacial pace. As ever, the slow march of progress in the healthcare system is put into stark relief when looking at other industries.

Today, millions of people manage their finances online. We can use apps to transfer money, pay for goods and services, apply for loans, research and make investments, exchange currencies and dabble in derivatives and cryptocurrencies. Collectively, we have the power to bring whole financial institutions to their knees through our individual actions. Or we can outsource our finances to accountants and investment managers.

Similarly, we can research holiday destinations, plan whole itineraries online, book flights, airport transfers, hire cars, hotels, restaurants and a wide range of activities on a smartphone. Or we can use a travel agent.

Technology-enabled change has transformed many industries

but it is worth noting that this has only happened since the start of the new millennium.

Why digital healthcare hasn't kept up

Contrast the above with the EHR systems used in most hospitals and health centres, which have hardly changed in four decades, and it surely raises some profound questions. Is managing our own healthcare really so different? Why have our healthcare systems not seen the revolutions that have taken place elsewhere?

There are broadly three answers to these questions. No, healthcare is not so different but it has lagged and we are about to see the revolution we have been waiting for, albeit a decade or more behind everyone else. Yes, healthcare is different because all the power is held by people and institutions that have a vested interest in maintaining the status quo. Yes, healthcare is different because, when it comes down to it, most patients don't actually want to take control of their own health and, for a variety of reasons mainly to do with psychological reassurance, prefer to subcontract this element of their lives to professionals.

The institutional inertia embedded in the health system is an interesting conundrum and possibly warrants a whole book of its own. Challenging it would involve exposing the power struggles that inherently take place between purchasers and providers of healthcare in the organisational structures that have evolved around the world, and ultimately the money that is lost in many of these health systems through inefficient and wasteful healthcare commissioning systems. Whether through insurance-based private medical systems that support a whole industry of intermediaries or a public healthcare commissioning system that is torn up and reinvented every few years just as it is starting to bed down and make real progress, a significant proportion of the money we invest in our healthcare systems does not make it to the front line where it can be used for direct patient care. And certainly the source of all this funding – ultimately the patients themselves – do not have control over how the money is spent. The irony is that many front-line clinicians – at least those who are more progressive – do not want the health system to be this way; they are equally trapped in the institutional structures we have inherited.

Why have patients not kept up?

The cultural shift required is not one that is solely in the hands of the healthcare professions, however. Patients need to play their part. It is telling that when healthcare organisations do provide access and an element of control to patients, the patients don't necessarily engage. This can't be due to technophobia; the same patients actively take part in online banking, shopping and various forms of social media. So, why is health different? I would suggest the following reasons.

- ❖ First, health records can be notoriously difficult to access; issues of data security tend to predominate in healthcare, but this can have the effect of putting patients off.
- ❖ Perhaps we haven't yet acclimatised to the idea that monitoring our health should be a much more regular pastime. It's something most of us do only sporadically.
- ❖ Healthcare events themselves can be quite sporadic, and deteriorating health can evolve with small, almost imperceptible changes over a long timeframe. Consequently, unlike other digital platforms requiring more regular engagement, healthcare is often something we dip in and out of.
- ❖ The elements we need to monitor health properly are not easily accessible. While people now have the means to easily monitor their heart rate, weight, BMI and blood pressure using readily obtainable and cost effective devices, wide-spectrum sampling of blood composition – at home – is not yet a thing. (Incidentally, this was why the promise of Theranos to do just that – which the company ultimately failed to deliver, resulting in its ultimate downfall – was so powerful. Though it would have saved the healthcare professions millions of dollars in radically more efficient testing, it also had the potential to put this element of health monitoring into the patients' hands). The above reasons all relate to patients in a relatively good state

of health; during an acute episode of care, however, many of these reasons don't apply. While you may not pay much attention to your health when you are fit and healthy, it can become your sole focus when you are not. You are suffering, you want to be well and you want to get back to full health as soon as possible. Events – you hope – will move much more quickly and you are incentivised to be involved in your care, not only to expedite your recovery, but also to understand what has happened, what your treatment options might be (there is rarely only one) along with their corresponding benefits and risks, and how you might prevent a recurrence. Moreover, you know recovery is usually not instant. You embark on a journey to get there, you want to monitor your progress on the way and you want to be able to maintain a dialogue about that progress and ask questions about things you don't understand. Despite this you can still be reluctant to take the initiative and become actively engaged.

While you are mostly happy to entrust your care to clinicians, you may, at one time or another, have wondered about people who have been in similar situations. What did they do? And what was the result? Has someone found a quick way out of this? And did they make a record somewhere that I can learn from? Can I google it? For this reason, the vast majority of people, I suspect, would also be willing – perhaps even wanting – with the right support and encouragement to contribute their experiences and perspectives into their care record if they were to be used – anonymously – to improve the experiences of similar patients in the future.

9 Clinical records – the next generation

With so many innovations starting to be adopted, emerging or on the horizon, digital and electronic health records (DHRs and EHRs) are poised for a significant transformation that will reshape healthcare delivery. After decades of seeing little significant progress in legacy systems, the next generation of these systems should finally move beyond mere digital documentation to become intelligent, interconnected platforms that actively support clinical decision making and patient engagement.

In many ways, this vision of the future will apply whether future health record systems consist of large monolithic EHRs or an ecosystem of DHRs working together to achieve the same goals. My preference is for the latter – I want every patient and clinician to have the best digital tools at their disposal – but if the previously outlined barriers to creating networks of interconnected best-of-breed systems are not overcome, then it is likely that this evolution may go in the former direction.

While the following sections summarise the advances you might expect to see (many of which were included in Chapter 3, if you didn't skip it), there are two basic things we need to get right before we can truly unlock the power of all the digital, technological and data advances at our disposal.

First, outcome measurement is key. We cannot collectively learn what works and what doesn't if we don't record it. We need to really challenge ourselves as to whether we are really recording outputs or inputs. Digital health records should start with the outcomes we are trying to achieve and work back from there.

Second, the structured care pathways I outlined in Chapter 8 are vital *today* in capturing patient journeys to allow comparisons to be made between the experiences (including outcomes) of one patient against another. I emphasise 'today' because the pace at which AI is advancing may soon allow patient journeys to be assembled and compared from very unstructured data, but that is not where we are now.

With these two essential pillars in place, we will then be in the best position to reap the benefits of all the technologies that are advancing over the horizon. Here, in summary, are the key developments you should expect to see in the coming years.

Intelligent and adaptive systems

AI-powered clinical decision support will become a cornerstone of next-generation EHRs. These systems will analyse patient data in real time against vast medical knowledge bases and provide contextually relevant, evidence-based suggestions to clinicians. For example, an EHR might alert a physician to a potential drug interaction or suggest an alternative treatment based on the latest clinical guidelines and the patient's unique medical history.

Predictive analytics will enable healthcare providers to identify at-risk patients before conditions worsen. By analysing patterns in vital signs, lab results, medication adherence and other data points, these systems will flag patients tending toward complications, allowing for earlier interventions. This proactive approach could dramatically reduce hospital readmissions and emergency department visits.

Natural language processing capabilities will transform unstructured clinical notes into structured, actionable data. Rather than forcing clinicians to navigate complex drop-down menus and checkboxes, which earlier I was promoting as an essential component to achieving the structured data necessary for data-driven healthcare, advanced NLP will allow clinicians to document naturally while the system automatically extracts and categorises relevant clinical information. This will significantly reduce documentation time while improving data quality.

Ambient clinical intelligence represents perhaps the most revolutionary advance and one that is already starting to be widely adopted. These systems will listen to patient–provider conversations and automatically document encounters, extracting key information about symptoms, diagnoses, treatment plans and follow-up instructions. This technology could eventually eliminate manual documentation entirely, allowing providers to focus completely on patient interaction.

Interoperability and integration

True interoperability between different healthcare systems and facilities will finally become a reality. Next-generation DHRs and EHRs will use standardised data formats and communication protocols to seamlessly exchange information, regardless of vendor or platform. This will eliminate information silos and ensure that providers have complete patient histories at their fingertips.

Seamless integration with patient-generated health data will bridge the gap between clinical visits. DHRs will incorporate data from patient devices such as blood pressure monitors, glucose meters, fitness trackers and smart scales, providing a more comprehensive view of health status over time rather than just snapshots during office visits.

API-first architectures will allow easier connections with specialised apps and services. Rather than attempting to build every possible feature into a monolithic system, even next-generation EHRs will function as platforms that third-party developers can build upon, creating purpose-built tools for specific clinical needs while maintaining data integration.

Integration with social determinants of health data from community resources will provide context beyond traditional medical information. Health record systems will incorporate data about housing status, food security, transportation access and other factors that significantly impact health outcomes, enabling more holistic care planning.

User experience improvements

More intuitive interfaces designed for specific clinical workflows will replace today's one-size-fits-all approaches. Cardiologists, emergency physicians and primary care providers have different information needs and work patterns; next-generation systems will recognise this and provide customised interfaces optimised for each speciality.

Reduced documentation burden through automation will address one of the primary complaints about current systems. Smart defaults, templated content that adapts to specific clinical scenarios and AI-assisted documentation will dramatically decrease the time providers spend entering data.

Mobile-first approaches will provide greater flexibility in care delivery. Rather than being tethered to workstations, clinicians will access complete system functionality on tablets, smartphones and other portable devices, allowing them to review information and document care wherever they are.

Customisable dashboards and information displays will present the most relevant information for different specialists. A nephrologist might see trending kidney function tests prominently displayed, while a psychiatrist might have medication history and mental status examination results prioritised in their view.

Data collection advances

Continuous monitoring through wearables and IoT medical devices will transform how we collect health data. Instead of periodic measurements during clinic visits, DHRs will incorporate streams of data from devices that monitor heart rate, activity levels, sleep patterns and other metrics continuously, providing a much more detailed picture of patient health.

Remote patient monitoring platforms integrated with central health record systems will enable virtual care at scale. Providers will be able to track patients with chronic conditions from afar, with automated alerts when measurements fall outside expected ranges. This will be particularly valuable for managing conditions such as heart failure, diabetes and hypertension.

Patient-reported outcomes collected via mobile apps between visits will add the patient's perspective to clinical data. Regular feedback on symptoms, functional status, quality of life and treatment side effects will help providers understand treatment effectiveness from the patient's viewpoint rather than relying solely on clinical measurements.

Genomic and phenotype data incorporated into patient records will enable truly personalised medicine. Next-generation EHRs will eventually store and interpret genetic information alongside traditional clinical data, allowing providers to select medications and treatments most likely to be effective based on a patient's genetic profile.

Environmental and behavioural data collection through smartphones and smart home devices will provide context for clinical findings. Information about air quality, activity patterns, sleep habits and dietary choices can help explain changes in health status and guide lifestyle interventions.

Data use innovations

Precision medicine approaches customised to individual patient characteristics will become standard practice. By integrating multiple data streams – clinical measurements, genetic information, environmental factors and more – systems will help clinicians tailor treatments to each patient's unique circumstances rather than following one-size-fits-all protocols.

Population health management tools will identify trends across patient groups, enabling more effective preventive care and resource allocation. Healthcare organisations will use DHR and EHR data to identify high-risk populations, track quality measures and implement targeted interventions to improve outcomes across communities.

Advanced visualisation of complex datasets will make clinical insights more accessible. Rather than presenting providers with pages of numbers and text, next-generation EHRs will use interactive graphics, heat maps and other visual tools to highlight patterns and trends that might otherwise go unnoticed.

Digital twins will model individual patient responses to treatments before they are administered. These computational models, built from a patient's comprehensive health data, will allow clinicians to simulate how different interventions might affect a specific individual, helping to select the optimal approach.

Federated learning systems will maintain privacy while enabling broader research use of health data. Rather than centralising sensitive information, these systems distribute the machine-learning process across multiple sites, with only the insights – not the raw data – being shared. This approach will accelerate medical research while protecting patient confidentiality.

The transformation of health record systems from passive documentation repositories to active clinical partners has the potential to be one of the most significant advances in healthcare technology. As these systems continue to evolve, the promise is that they will reduce clinician burnout, improve clinical outcomes, enhance the patient experience and ultimately deliver on the promise of data-driven healthcare.

10 Challenges to adoption

We are on the verge of a potential sea change in how we manage patients through their healthcare journeys. With a wide array of new digital technologies and data analysis capabilities, the opportunities to improve healthcare service efficiency and effectiveness are greater than ever. In particular, the potential to finally introduce data-driven healthcare as standard stands teasingly on the threshold of our new digital healthcare landscape. So, why might it not happen? What possible reasons can be put forward for not jumping in with both feet?

Affordability

Let's start with the obvious one. Leading-edge technologies are not cheap and health services are cash strapped. The demands being placed on our healthcare systems today far outweigh the pace at which additional funding can be made available. This creates a frustrating catch-22 where the substantial cost savings and improved outcomes promised by new digital and data technologies can't be accessed without a significant injection of cash that healthcare organisations simply do not have. While seed funding for the development of new technologies is often in plentiful supply (depending on the economic cycle), the seed capital for deployment in live clinical environments isn't, especially where the new technology has no track record.

Healthcare managers recognise this problem but the solution isn't always clear. However, if new technologies come hand in hand with robust business cases demonstrating the expected benefits of adoption, it is often not expensive to run a pilot and test the claims prior to a wider roll-out.

Data and communication standards

Despite many valiant attempts to standardise healthcare data, not just in-country but internationally, very few of these have stood the test of time. Whichever system or set of protocols rises to be the latest would-be king of standards, it is inevitably replaced by something supposedly better. Healthcare providers consequently find it hard to keep up with the changing landscape and can often be several incarnations behind.

This problem is exacerbated by legacy systems that are hard to shift in favour of newer, more up-to-date regimes. Organisations that have invested many years in collecting data to a previous national or international standard are understandably reluctant to sacrifice the longitudinal benefit and start again. A new data standard might be an improvement but it can take many years to collect enough data to really reap the rewards.

To a certain extent the issue can be alleviated by mapping old to new coding systems – and this does happen – but the real trick is to perform this work at an international level (eg within the World Health Organization) and plan the design to be as flexible and expandable as possible. I would hope we have learned enough lessons historically that future proofing new coding systems for longevity is now a real possibility.

I demonstrated how powerful the analysis of care pathways could be in heralding a sea change in the development of effective and efficient services, especially when combined with outcome data, just as I also noted the importance of adopting standards for reporting and data exchange. The benefits of data-driven healthcare approaches cannot be maximised without healthcare organisations collaborating with commissioners and other providers to agree common protocols and frameworks for data to allow systematic recording. Artificial intelligence may begin to help us sift through the patchy quagmire that currently exists in data capture but a lot more could be achieved if we could help it too.

And data standardisation does not mean a reduction in personalisation, a common misconception that presents an additional challenge. In fact, the opposite is true. The more we can standardise existing data, and the more types of new data we can provide in a standardised form, the more we are able to provide patients with a truly personalised experience.

Privacy and confidentiality

Medical records contain highly sensitive information including diagnoses, treatment plans, medication histories and personal identifiers that require robust safeguards. When considering new systems, healthcare providers must balance the potential benefits of technological advancement against their ethical and legal obligations to protect patient confidentiality, specifically evaluating whether these technologies can consistently maintain data integrity while preventing unauthorised access, modification or deletion. The potential consequences of inadequate protection – ranging from compromised patient care to legal liability – can create barriers to adoption, particularly for technologies that lack an established track record as a secure data repository.

Another significant factor is the complex regulatory environment surrounding medical data protection. Healthcare institutions must navigate strict compliance requirements such as HIPAA in the United States, GDPR in Europe and various national and regional frameworks worldwide. New technologies must demonstrate comprehensive compliance with these regulations, including features for access controls, audit trails, encryption standards and breach notification protocols. The costs of implementing these protective measures, training staff and maintaining ongoing compliance often outweigh perceived benefits of new systems, especially when existing solutions, though perhaps less efficient, already meet regulatory standards. This regulatory burden particularly impacts smaller healthcare providers with limited resources for compliance management and risk assessment.

The threat of hefty fines, reputational damage and erosion of patient trust in the event of a data breach, also makes healthcare providers cautious about adopting new systems without robust security measures and clear protocols for data handling. Together, these concerns create a tension between innovation and the fundamental healthcare principle of 'first, do no harm' when it comes to patient data protection.

My personal view is that the use of *anonymised* patient data to inform research and data-driven healthcare should be part of the contract between a patient and their healthcare provider. With such an agreement in place, the value locked up in each patient record can be used to benefit other patients without risking breaches of privacy and confidentiality.

Cyber security

Heightened concerns about cybersecurity could present another barrier. The healthcare sector is an increasingly attractive target for cybercriminals, with electronic health records containing comprehensive personal, financial and medical information that commands premium prices on illicit markets. The potential consequences of a successful cyberattack on patient record systems are severe, ranging from the theft and misuse of confidential information to the disruption of critical healthcare services and even risks to patient safety. The healthcare sector's documented history of ransomware attacks, data breaches and system compromises creates understandable caution, particularly when evaluating solutions with limited security track records or those utilising emerging technologies without established security frameworks.

Moreover, the interconnected nature of modern healthcare systems, with numerous devices, networks and third-party vendors, expands the attack surface and creates more potential vulnerabilities. Outdated legacy systems, which are often deeply embedded in healthcare workflows, can be particularly susceptible to cyber threats. The challenge of securing these complex environments, coupled with the increasing sophistication of cyberattacks, makes healthcare organisations cautious about adopting new technologies that might introduce additional security risks.

A lack of cybersecurity skills and resources exacerbates the problem. Implementing new patient record technologies requires not just the initial deployment but ongoing security monitoring, vulnerability management, patch implementation and incident response capabilities. Many healthcare organisations, particularly smaller clinics and rural hospitals, lack dedicated cybersecurity personnel and struggle to compete for qualified security professionals against better-resourced industries. This resource constraint often leads to risk-averse decision making where organisations maintain legacy systems with known but manageable security limitations rather than introducing new technologies that would require additional cybersecurity investments and expertise that may be beyond their current capabilities.

Unfortunately, defending against the potential threat of cyberattacks from bad actors is now part of the cost of operating in this field. It is an expensive business – especially when compared against all the healthcare that could be provided with the same funding – but the ramifications of a successful attack are often catastrophic for all concerned and we really have no alternative than to provide the same protection to patient data as we would to nuclear reactors.

Patient safety

Aside from the cybersecurity impact on patient safety, other patient safety concerns could impede the adoption of new healthcare technologies. I have already discussed the importance of healthcare providers prioritising patient wellbeing above all else in adopting new clinical support systems, and any perceived risk of harm associated with a new technology can create substantial resistance. Today, this is particularly true of new technologies employing AI, where patient safety concerns are a significant barrier to adoption. Until an AI system can be shown not to hallucinate (where it interprets the data available to it incorrectly), there will continue to be a concern that AI will give bad advice, possibly leading to patient harm.

Additionally, the integration of new record systems with existing clinical technologies presents substantial patient safety challenges. Modern healthcare relies on a complex ecosystem of interconnected devices and systems. New patient record technologies must demonstrate reliable interoperability with critical systems while maintaining data integrity across all interfaces.

Similarly, if healthcare professionals find a new technology difficult to use or if it disrupts their ability to provide timely and effective care, they may be unwilling to adopt it, hindering the potential for improved patient record management and overall healthcare delivery.

These risks create understandable hesitation, particularly when new technologies lack extensive real-world testing across diverse healthcare environments or when implementation requires substantial workflow changes that could introduce unfamiliar errors during the transition period. System downtime, data corruption or interface errors in newer technologies lacking a track record might prevent clinicians from accessing critical information during emergencies or cause treatment delays when historical records are unavailable. If a new system is perceived to introduce the potential for errors in medication administration, misidentification of patients or loss of critical data, medical professionals would be hesitant to embrace it.

Legacy systems at least have the benefit of being tried and tested over time with any identified patient safety issues designed out long before. The fear of causing adverse events, even if a new technology promises long-term benefits, can lead to a preference to remain on these familiar, albeit less efficient, legacy systems.

Like cyber security, prioritising patient safety in system design is now part of the cost of doing business in healthcare technology. Developing patient safety test suites alongside application software development can ensure that it is impossible for patients to get lost in the system while also enabling unusual scenarios to be simulated to mitigate against patients suffering adverse events even in edge cases. This requires more investment at the development stage but is essential if the 'first, do no harm' principle of serving patients well is to be maintained.

Patient demand

Patients are increasingly active participants in their healthcare, and their expectations and preferences can drive or hinder the uptake of new systems. Many patients, particularly older adults or those with limited technological fluency, express anxiety about the increasing digitisation of healthcare and may resist changes to how their information is managed. They worry about losing the personal touch of traditional doctor–patient relationships or fear being unable to navigate patient portals. While, on the one hand, they may push for technologies that enhance joined-up care and provide seamless access to their records, they are also prominent in expressing concerns about user interfaces and data protection and privacy. These divergent patient expectations can create complex adoption hurdles.

Furthermore, concerns about the digital divide and health equity can also play a role. Some patients may lack the necessary technological literacy or access to devices and internet connectivity, creating disparities in their ability to engage with new digital health tools. Healthcare providers may be hesitant to adopt technologies that could exacerbate these inequalities or alienate vulnerable patient populations. The resources required for patient education, providing technical support and maintaining alternative access options for those unable or unwilling to use new systems could delay or complicate the adoption process. This delicate balancing act between innovation and inclusivity might lead healthcare providers to proceed cautiously with adopting radically innovative technological change.

In reality, excluding minority groups who have no access to digital healthcare options is not going to suppress the inevitable rise of new technologies. And nor should it. I am surprised at how often new technologies are held back because they are not inclusive of one group or another because most of the time the impact is the opposite of what patient advocates fear. If the majority of patients are able to take advantage of digital automation then this provides more human capacity to provide better and more personalised services for the disadvantaged and hard-to-reach communities.

Data volumes

Earlier, I identified a wide range of emerging technologies that are poised for adoption across the healthcare community. Whether the accumulation of ever more 1s and 0s arises from higher-resolution medical imaging, continuous patient-monitoring devices, genomic sequencing or unstructured clinical notes pouring into patient records from ambient listening technology, the sheer amount of patient data associated with these is growing exponentially. This expansion serves only to extend the concerns already expressed around privacy and cybersecurity; larger volumes of data create more significant risks of breaches.

But migrating, storing, managing and analysing these vast datasets will also require robust and scalable infrastructure, which can be costly and complex to implement. The costs associated with data storage, increased network bandwidth requirements and expanded back-up systems to accommodate growing data volumes, further complicate the business case for new technologies.

These concerns are particularly pronounced for rural or under-resourced healthcare facilities that may lack the technical infrastructure to support data-intensive applications, creating a technological divide that can exacerbate healthcare disparities. Yet once again, the benefits of technological adoption far outweigh the (hopefully temporary) disparities that might arise. And this will be exponentially true once AI gets its claws into the data. We haven't even begun to appreciate what AI might discover when let loose on oceans of patient records but I'm confident it will find so many valuable insights that the costs of collecting and storing the data will be eclipsed by the benefits.

Barriers to entry

Providers of new digital healthcare technology often struggle to gain entry into the market. One major hurdle is the complex regulatory landscape, including stringent data privacy laws and other region-specific regulations. Healthcare's highly regulated environment demands extensive compliance documentation, certification processes and security validations that can stretch development timelines and drain start-up capital. Regulatory hurdles create asymmetric advantages for established vendors with existing compliance frameworks and institutional knowledge, effectively pricing many innovative start-ups out of the market before they can demonstrate their technological superiority. The substantial investment in secure infrastructure and compliance measures required can be particularly challenging for smaller start-ups with limited resources.

Additionally, healthcare's deeply entrenched procurement practices and risk-averse institutional culture create substantial commercial obstacles. Healthcare organisations typically prioritise vendors with established track records, extensive reference sites and demonstrable financial stability to ensure long-term support for mission-critical systems. New entrants struggle to overcome this 'credibility gap' without prior healthcare deployments, creating a paradoxical situation where providers can't win contracts without references but can't build references without contracts.

Another key barrier is the challenge of integrating new technologies with existing, often outdated, electronic health record (EHR) systems. Interoperability issues, lack of standardised data formats and the need for seamless data exchange can create significant technical hurdles. Suppliers of legacy systems may also feel threatened by newer vendors and technologies and consequently hinder cooperation, sensing they might be turkeys voting for Christmas.

Furthermore, healthcare providers may be hesitant to adopt new technologies due to concerns about the cost of implementation, training staff and potential disruption to their workflow. The long sales cycles and the need to demonstrate clear ROI in terms of improved patient outcomes or cost savings often result in new entrants to the market not getting their product off the ground. Implementing new systems in a live clinical environment can also be fraught with risk and it isn't as if public-sector IT disasters are unknown.

Today, it is very rare for a supplier to enter the market with a new digital healthcare record. Given all the challenges identified in this chapter so far, the cost of getting a credible product to market is almost always prohibitive to new entrants. Even if a new company was to tick all the regulatory, security, confidentiality and patient safety boxes, replicating and bettering the range of functionality provided by legacy systems takes significant time and money. Anyone investing in such an undertaking – even though it is desperately needed – will require deep pockets and lots of patience, not a common feature of our current corporate world.

There are potentially two white knights that could solve this conundrum. The first – the option taken by most new entrants – is to build something very simple that does what it does better than anything else, and once established alongside other systems, gradually increase the functionality over time to eventually usurp an incumbent. The second is AI: if the promise that AI will eventually develop software as well – or better – than humans comes to pass, then it will inevitably create a paradigm shift in application design and almost certainly accelerate the pace of development exponentially.

Digital skills

As a general rule, if people in the caring professions were as interested in data and digital technologies as they are in looking after their patients, then they would have selected a different career. There is a global shortage of technical skills and as a result salaries in the tech sector tend to be higher than in healthcare, with bigger salaries achievable at a younger age. Medical, clinical and therapeutic disciplines are collectively known as the caring professions for a reason. And while many might choose to commit to years of intense study for a whole variety of reasons, healthcare professionals mostly choose their careers because – that's right – they care about the health and wellbeing of their fellow human beings.

Passion for all things digital and data driven, then, is not unknown in the healthcare profession, but it is rare. Midway through the past decade, the NHS in England launched its Global Digital Exemplar (GDE) programme, investing almost £400 million in a handful of healthcare organisations that were internationally recognised to be delivering improvements in the quality of care, through the world-class use of digital technologies and information. The aim behind the programme was to encourage these trusts to get even further ahead of the digital curve and then transfer their knowledge and learning to less digitally enabled organisations, potentially globally. But at least one large trust, after an extensive assessment of its internal IT capabilities, came to the conclusion that its GDE funding would be best spent on improving the Microsoft Office skills (think Word, Excel) of its front-line staff. Such is the gap between the technologies now available and the availability of skills to use it.

New digital technologies, then, may expose the lack of proficiency needed to reap the benefits of adoption, and may require substantial investment in retraining across all personnel who interact with it, including doctors, nurses, administrative staff and allied health professionals. This can lead to resistance to change, decreased efficiency and an increased risk of errors. It is certainly not unknown for staff who are not adequately trained to navigate a new clinical support system to revert to less efficient paper-based methods, undermining the original purpose of the digital upgrade. All of these challenges become particularly acute in settings already experiencing staffing shortages or high turnover rates, where training resources are stretched thin and institutional knowledge is regularly lost.

The digital skills concern extends beyond basic operational competency to more nuanced aspects of healthcare technology use. Healthcare workers must develop sufficient digital discernment to recognise when systems are functioning correctly, identify potential errors or anomalies in data presentation, and understand the limitations of automated recommendations. This level of technical sophistication requires ongoing education beyond initial implementation training, creating sustained operational costs and potential resistance from practitioners concerned about technology diminishing their clinical autonomy. Upskilling clinicians in data analysis techniques would help, but this would require even more investment and risk becoming a distraction from providing direct clinical care.

This challenge will partially solve itself as younger generations – already pre-wired to use digital technologies – move into the workforce. Better, more usable and intuitive software will also help, as will AI as it closes the gap between human and machine understanding. Today, I don't need to know how to use a word processor to write a letter; I can just ask an AI tool to do it for me.

Keeping up with technology advances

Patient record systems – particularly EHRs – represent major capital investments that typically require five- to ten-year implementation and optimisation cycles before delivering their full clinical and financial benefits. In a world where technology heralds a new generation every three years, mobile phones last 18 months and browser software is refreshed several times a year, this extended timeline creates significant misalignment with the pace of technological evolution. Consequently, organisations fear investing millions in solutions that may become outdated before achieving positive returns, and often even before they go live.

The risk of technological obsolescence is particularly concerning when considering emerging technologies such as cloud platforms, AI-enhanced workflows or interoperability standards that continue evolving rapidly. Decision makers often delay adoption while waiting for the technology landscape to stabilise, creating a perpetual cycle of postponement as each new innovation wave introduces fresh uncertainty. In today's world, that day will never come. If anything, the level of technological instability is only going to increase.

The operational burden of continual technological adaptation further compounds adoption challenges. Healthcare providers must maintain clinical operations while implementing increasingly frequent software updates, security patches and feature enhancements. Each change necessitates workflow adjustments, staff retraining and validation testing to ensure patient safety is not compromised. The cumulative effect creates 'upgrade fatigue', with practitioners growing resistant to learning perpetually changing interfaces and administrators struggling to budget for ongoing implementation support. Smaller healthcare organisations face particular difficulties sustaining the technical expertise and change-management resources needed to keep pace with technology evolution.

It is therefore not surprising that stability is often prioritised over innovation, maintaining outdated but functional systems rather than embracing potentially superior but rapidly evolving technologies whose long-term support models and upgrade pathways remain uncertain.

So, yes, the introduction and widespread adoption of data-driven healthcare is not without its challenges, but can we honestly envision a future world that does not have it as a fundamental component of how we do healthcare in the future? I can't. And if it is inevitable that it will one day come to pass, as I believe it must, then we may as well start tackling the challenges now. With so much at stake, there is no time like the present.

11 Conclusion – the future is bright

Today, digital technologies are revolutionising the way medical records are created, stored and utilised in healthcare. Beyond the basic transition from paper to electronic health records (EHRs), advanced innovations such as natural language processing, blockchain security, cloud-based systems and AI-powered analytics are transforming patient data into dynamic tools for improved care. Mobile applications now allow patients to access and contribute to their own health information, while interoperability standards enable seamless sharing between different healthcare systems. These technologies not only streamline documentation and reduce administrative burden but also have the potential to unlock new capabilities in predictive medicine, personalised treatment planning and population health management – turning what was once a static repository of information into an intelligent ecosystem that enhances clinical decision making and patient outcomes.

With a newly charged focus on outcome measurement and structured clinical pathways – the two key foundational pillars that will make all this work to best effect – I believe the reality of true, data-driven healthcare could just be around the corner. Finally, as patients, we will not only be able to seek the opinion and advice of the one healthcare professional that comes to our aid, but potentially a myriad of experiences derived from both experts and other patients with lived experience who have trodden this path before us. Through data-driven healthcare we will all be able to supplement recommendations for tried-and-tested treatments, backed by clinical trials, with the wisdom of the crowd, assessing the healthcare journeys and outcomes of potentially thousands of people who have gone before us, many of whom may have even successfully found more natural, alternative treatments to prevailing Western medicine. The point is, patients will have all the treatment options available, together with their prognoses for a successful outcome, allowing them to make informed choices. Sometimes these will balance benefits and risks, such as side effects, but in the future healthcare landscape, transparency will become king.

None of this can happen, of course, unless healthcare organisations keep investing in new digital technologies. Despite the challenges and concerns around privacy, cybersecurity, patient safety and digital skills I outlined in the previous chapter, healthcare organisations should not be deterred from adopting new digital technologies. The prize is too big to be ignored and we are already way behind. The long-term benefits of these technologies, including improved patient outcomes, increased efficiency and enhanced data analysis, outweigh the short-term challenges. Delaying adoption could lead to missed opportunities for innovation and leave organisations lagging further behind in an increasingly digital healthcare landscape. If improving efficiency and outcomes isn't incentive enough, then perhaps FOMO needs to be the new watchword.

So many aspects of our lives today are data driven, from the TV shows we watch to the books we read and the products we buy, whether we are aware of it or not. In healthcare, being data driven should not in any sense be seen as being radical. It should just be.

References

AIHW (2024) 'Health expenditure Australia 2022–3'. URL: www.aihw.gov.au/reports/health-welfare-expenditure/health-expenditure-australia-2022-23/contents/overview/total-health-spending

Ananth, V (2024) 'Digital twins – fast-tracking the future of healthcare'. *Journal of mHealth* 28 August. URL: thejournalofmhealth.com/digital-twins-fast-tracking-the-future-of-healthcare

Barnfield, K (2022) 'Heart transplant waiting list increases by 85% in 10 years'. Sky News. URL: news.sky.com/story/they-gave-me-a-week-to-live-heart-transplant-waiting-list-increases-by-85-in-10-years-12541659

Burton, C R, Williams, L et al (2021) 'Theory and practical guidance for effective de-implementation of practices across health and care services: A realist synthesis'. *Health and Social Care Delivery Research* 9(2). URL: www.journalslibrary.nihr.ac.uk/hsdr/HSDR09020

BusinessWire (2025) 'Telehealth and telemedicine research, 2020–2024 & 2025–2030'. URL: www.businesswire.com/news/home/20250110337200/en/Telehealth-and-Telemedicine-Research-2020-2024-2025-2030-with-Analyst-Recommendations---Integration-of-Wearable-Devices-and-the-IoT-Develop-Strategies-for-Expanding-Adoption-in-Emerging-Markets---ResearchAndMarkets.com

Carding, N (2021) 'NHS needs to "radically simplify" data sharing rules, says tech chief'. *Health Service Journal* 28 September.

Cartan Capital (2023) 'The wearable revolution'. URL: www.linkedin.com/pulse/wearable-revolution-cartancapital-lo1fe

Economist (2017) 'The world's most valuable resource is no longer oil, but data'. *The Economist.* URL: www.economist.com/leaders/2017/05/06/the-worlds-most-valuable-resource-is-no-longer-oil-but-data

Gawande, A (2009) *The Checklist Manifesto: How to get things right.* Profile.

Henderson, H (2024) 'CRISPR clinical trials: A 2024 update'. Innovative Genomics. URL: innovativegenomics.org/news/crispr-clinical-trials-2024

Hoeksma, J (2016) 'CSUS: Big differences in usability of clinical software'. *Digital Health.* URL: www.digitalhealth.net/2016/06/csus-big-differences-in-usability-of-clinical-software

Jia, Y, Wang, W et al (2018) 'Perceived user preferences and usability evaluation of mainstream wearable devices for health monitoring'. *PeerJ Life & Environment* 25/7/18.

Johns Hopkins Medicine (2024) 'Brian–computer interface studies'. URL: www.hopkinsmedicine.org/neurology-neurosurgery/clinical-trials/brain-computer-interface

King's Fund, The (2022) 'NHS trusts in deficit'. URL: www.kingsfund.org.uk/insight-and-analysis/data-and-charts/nhs-trusts-deficit

Mayden (2022) 'NHS EPR Usability Survey results: what is iaptus? And how did we do?' URL: iaptus.co.uk/2022/09/nhs-epr-usability-survey-results-what-is-iaptus-and-how-did-we-do

Meskó, B (2017) 'What could you do with cheap genome sequencing now?' URL: www.linkedin.com/pulse/what-could-you-do-cheap-genome-sequencing-now-bertalan-meskó-md-phd

Milmo, D (2025) 'Microsoft says AI system better than doctors at diagnosing complex health conditions'. *Guardian* 30 June. URL: www.theguardian.com/technology/2025/jun/30/microsoft-ai-system-better-doctors-diagnosing-health-conditions-research

Moore, J (2024) 'How to harness the power of health data to improve patient outcomes'. World Economic Forum. URL:

www.weforum.org/stories/2024/01/how-to-harness-health-data-to-improve-patient-outcomes-wef24

Mount Sinai (2025) 'Personalized cancer vaccine proves promising in a phase 1 trial at Mount Sinai'. URL: www.mountsinai.org/about/newsroom/2025/personalized-cancer-vaccine-proves-promising-in-a-phase-1-trial-at-mount-sinai

NAO (2011) 'The National Programme for IT in the NHS: An update on the delivery of detailed care records systems'. URL: www.nao.org.uk/reports/the-national-programme-for-it-in-the-nhs-an-update-on-the-delivery-of-detailed-care-records-systems

Nuance (2022) 'Assessing the burden of clinical documentation'. URL: www.nuance.com/asset/en_uk/collateral/enterprise/report/rpt-assessing-the-burden-of-clinical-documentation-en-uk.pdf

Odeh, V A, Chen, Y et al (2024) 'Recent advances in the wearable devices for monitoring and management of heart failure'. *Reviews in Cardiovascular Medicine* 25(10).

ONS (2017) 'What affects an area's healthy life expectancy?' URL: www.ons.gov.uk/peoplepopulationandcommunity/healthandsocialcare/healthandlifeexpectancies/articles/whataffectsanareashealthylifeexpectancy/2017-06-28

ONS (2018) 'Overview of the UK population: November 2018'. URL: www.ons.gov.uk/peoplepopulationandcommunity/populationandmigration/populationestimates/articles/overviewoftheukpopulation/november2018

Pfleger, S G, Haertel, M E M & Plentz, P D M (2025) 'UV-C disinfection robots: A systematic review'. *Journal of Field Robotics* 8 May. URL: onlinelibrary.wiley.com/doi/10.1002/rob.22555

RBC Capital Markets (2025) 'The healthcare data explosion'. URL: www.rbccm.com/en/gib/healthcare/episode/the_healthcare_data_explosion

Richter, F (2023) 'Charted: How life expectancy is changing around the world'. World Economic Forum. URL: www.weforum.org/stories/2023/02/charted-how-life-expectancy-is-changing-around-the-world

Swayne, M (2025) 'Quantum computing helps design new cancer drug candidates'. Quantum Insider. URL: thequantuminsider.com/2025/01/23/quantum-computing-helps-design-new-cancer-drug-candidates

Syed, M (2015) *Black Box Thinking: Growth mindset and the secrets of high performance*. John Murray.

Tariq, R A, Vashisht, R et al (2024) 'Medication dispensing errors and prevention'. StatPearls. URL: www.ncbi.nlm.nih.gov/books/NBK519065

Trustmarque (2025) 'Smart hospitals: Transforming patient care in the NHS'. URL: trustmarque.com/resources/smart-hospitals-transforming-patient-care-in-the-nhs

WHO (2008) 'Safe surgery saves lives'. URL: iris.who.int/bitstream/handle/10665/70080/WHO_IER_PSP_2008.07_eng.pdf

Acknowledgements

It has been my dream for a long time to mine the gold in patient data and put it to good use. In fact, that was the founding purpose of Mayden when the company first came into existence 25 years ago.

So I first have to acknowledge the thousands of clinicians who, every day, pour volumes of data into their clinical management systems knowing they will never see most of it ever again.

But there are a few people I would want to acknowledge specifically and without whom this book would probably never have seen the light of day.

Stephen Bridge, former CEO of Papworth Hospital, who brought me into the health sector and facilitated my introduction to healthcare data.

Bruce Finnamore, who gave me further wide-ranging opportunities to play with healthcare data in a variety of settings while building a great consultancy practice and offering many words of wisdom along the way.

Chris Ward and Ruth Bridgeman, for believing in me and providing the funding that allowed us to work the data magic and support the transformation of cancer care in England.

Special thanks must go to Professor David Clark who, in recognising the data problem, established a new psychological therapy service in England founded on the principles of continuous outcome measurement and stepped care pathways, and in doing so provided an open door for me to step through and demonstrate that the principles set out in this book are not just a pipe dream but the basis of an approach to healthcare that is recognised as world-class around the globe.

And equally to Doctor Ben Wright without whose vision, faith, support and appetite for risk, the digital systems we developed in resonance with this dream would never have existed.

Finally, to the Right Book Company team, without whose perennial professionalism this book would have never evolved from a motley collection of slides and quickly forgotten conference talks into something enduring.

I am forever grateful to you all.

About the author

Chris May is the founder of Mayden, a leading healthcare technology company based in Bath, UK. With over three decades of experience in the healthcare sector, he has established himself as a prominent figure in health tech innovation and digital transformation and was recognised as one of the Top 50 most ambitious business leaders by LDC and *The Times* in 2022.

Chris's core philosophy centres on the belief that healthcare should be constantly improving and that data and technology are key drivers of these improvements. This has shaped Mayden's approach to developing practical, clinician-focused solutions, and is a big motivator for the writing of this book.

In addition to his work at Mayden, he also established the iO Academy, a software training school, to help address a local tech skills gap across Bath and Bristol. The academy produced over one thousand graduates and was independently assessed as the sixth best in the world.

Chris is a published author of both fiction and non-fiction. His first non-fiction title, *Made Without Managers*, was awarded a Highly Commended accolade at the UK Business Book Awards. His novels, *Silent Light* and *The Son of Man*, are mystery thrillers set in the near future.

EU Safety Representative: euComply OÜ Pärnu mnt 139b-14 11317 Tallinn
Estonia hello@eucompliancepartner.com +33 756 90241

www.ingramcontent.com/pod-product-compliance
Lightning Source LLC
Chambersburg PA
CBHW040521220526
45473CB00013B/2940